Lifelines

to
Cancer Survival

A New Approach to
Personalized Care

Published by

IMP Integrative Medicine Publishing
P.O. Box 1817
Royal Oak, MI 48076
www.LifelinestoCancerSurvival.com

Editor: Ilene Stankiewicz
Cover design and layout: Deborah Perdue, Ilumination Graphics

First Printing

Publisher's Cataloging-in-Publication Data

Roby, Mark.
   Lifelines to cancer survival : a new approach to personalized care /
by Mark Roby, PA-C.

        pages ; cm

   Includes bibliographical references.
   ISBN: 978-0-9861673-0-0 (softcover)
   ISBN: 978-0-9861673-1-7 (Mobi)
   ISBN: 978-0-9861673-2-4 (EPUB)

   1. Cancer—Patient—Care. 2. Cancer—Alternative treatment.
3. Cancer—Diet therapy. 4. Cancer—Patients—Attitudes. 5. Personalized medicine.
6. Holistic medicine. I. Title.

RC262 .R63 2015
616.994

Lifelines

to
Cancer Survival

A New Approach to
Personalized Care

Mark Roby, PA-C

IMP

INTEGRATIVE MEDICINE PUBLISHING

This book is dedicated to:

Kathleen, the love of my life
Without your love and support, I would not be alive.

Ruth Betty, my mom
Thank you for the wonderful life you gave me.
Your guidance has meant so much
and your prayers have sustained me.

In Gratitude

I wish to thank the staffs at the following institutions/organizations* for their devoted care and support during my fight for survival. So many people helped and made all the difference, including doctors, nurses, social workers, technicians, aides, and even custodial staffs. They all contributed to my recovery and remission, for which I am eternally grateful.

These include:

• Cleveland Clinic (Cleveland, Ohio)

• Columbia Presbyterian Hospital (New York City)

• Henry Ford Health System (metro Detroit)

• Northwestern Memorial Hospital (Chicago)

• William Beaumont Hospital (Royal Oak, Michigan)

• NYU Langone Medical Center (New York City)

• Mount Sinai Hospital (New York City)

• Attitudinal Healing International (100 centers, including metro Detroit)

• The Hope Lodge/American Cancer Society

*A portion of this book's proceeds will be donated to these institutions/organizations.

Contents

Foreword

*T*here are many books that have been written about cancer. But for me, the best books by far, are those written from the heart by people who have actually experienced cancer first-hand.

This deeply moving book, *Lifelines to Cancer Survival*, by Mark Roby is a dramatic, personal adventure about someone who was told 12 years ago that he had just a few months to live, and that there was nothing that anyone could do to prevent the cancer from worsening, much less cure it. Even in the face of dire predictions, Mark faced some of his toughest challenges with unlimited hope, love, and enthusiasm for life.

I first met Mark after he read my book, *Love Is Letting Go of Fear*. In 1986 he phoned me regarding a friend of his who was dying in a hospital. I later invited Mark to come out to California to attend a workshop in Attitudinal Healing. It was about a year later that he and Laurie Pappas helped start the Metro Detroit Center for Attitudinal Healing in Detroit, Michigan. Since that time, we have become close friends. We've talked and emailed each other throughout the years. Mark not only became my close friend, he also became my teacher.

Mark has come close to death several times. I remember a day when his fear was climbing the ladder, and I suggested that he might want to choose to live in a different consciousness. When one is in a consciousness of helping and loving another person, fear starts to disappear. He followed my suggestion, and in an amazing way his fear started to disappear.

After reading my book, he became a student of *A Course in Miracles*. One of his morning rituals became a prayer from the *Course*. It goes like this:

> I am not a body.
> I am free.
> For I am still
> As God created me.

In addition, he watched and rewatched videos of TV programs in which I had been interviewed, along with children who had catastrophic illnesses. In these programs, I shared the concepts of attitudinal healing that I'd taught these children, and many of them went on to survive into adulthood. As Mark started to see his own identity beyond the limitations of a physical body, as a spiritual being, much of his fear dissolved. This amazing man has told me that he feels he would have been dead years ago had he not started to focus on living a spiritual life and finding another way of looking at the world and his body.

Along the way, Mark had a liver transplant. He also began to change his belief system into one where he believed that *nothing was impossible*. He chose not to be a victim or to complain. He learned he could be peaceful and happy, regardless of what was happening to his body. And he identified with some of the morning rituals that my wife Diane and I perform, like:

> We decide each morning to make this day the best and happiest day of our lives, regardless of what is put on our plates, and regardless of the state of our body.

> Today, I am determined to have no thoughts or attitudes that are hurtful to others or to myself.

Throughout our long friendship, Mark has told me the Principle of Attitudinal Healing that he particularly relates to is "Health is inner peace. Healing is the letting go of fear."

Then, he met an extraordinary woman by the name of Kathleen. She became the love of Mark's life. Together, they have navigated many difficult journeys and have been amazing helpers to countless others who have sought Mark's guidance. He is becoming adept at integrative medicine and cancer survival, not only to help himself but to help others. In this book, he breaks down the long process that was involved in learning cancer survival strategies. These are the strategies that have become "lifelines" for Mark and other cancer survivors.

Besides understanding the importance of letting go of fear, Mark now has an unshakable belief that your thoughts can change your reality. As you change your mind, you invariably experience the world differently, and you change your life. A major part of the new mindset is letting go of the hurt of past transgressions. As forgiveness became part of his heartbeat, Mark healed his relationships.

If you are looking for someone to inspire you, you have picked the right author to read. I know in my heart that you will be nourished as I have been from the courage and helpful attitudes he has demonstrated throughout all his challenges. Mark, you have brilliantly demonstrated the power of love over fear in life, and I love and congratulate you for that.

Gerald Jampolsky, MD
Founder, Attitudinal Healing
www.ahinternational.org

Preface

*I*n late March of 2003, I was lying in a large, cavernous chemo room in Michigan. As 10 million units of interferon coursed into me, I could feel myself going into the abyss. Even though I was in this dream state, I can remember my oncologist whispering in my ear, "Mark, why are you going all around the country looking for answers? There aren't any. This interferon isn't going to work; neither is Avastin®, thalidomide, or even a clinical trial drug. Why can't you accept the inevitable? You'll be gone in the next three to four months."

I couldn't believe what he was saying to me. I was in shock and disbelief. I thought his job was to save my life! I said to myself, "What are these doctors telling their patients?" The physician who was assigned to help save my life seemed ready to give up. I became madder than hell. Over time, I turned that anger into action.

I never want to forget that moment. Why? Because it was a turning point for me. I never want any other patient to hear what I heard or feel what I felt like when that doctor gave me a death sentence. I know what it's like to be in *your* shoes, given a grim prognosis and no hope. That's why I wrote this book.

The sole purpose of *Lifelines* is to increase patients' survival times, *your* survival time, especially if you are facing rare, aggressive, or advanced malignancies. *Lifelines to Cancer Survival* offers you, the reader, cutting-edge, real-time research and tools that you will not find compiled in one resource anywhere else.

When I was hit with cancer, there was no handbook or roadmap on how to survive it. This book is a compilation of a decade's worth of research and personal insight that

I have gained to keep myself alive. The media loves to herald successful cancer patients as heroes. I am no hero, but I know what it takes to survive. It is my hope that these life-saving tools will empower you in your own journey with cancer.

Introduction

It's no coincidence that you picked up this book. Your will to live and intuition brought you here. With a medical insider's knowledge of what it takes to stay alive when all the odds are against you, *Lifelines to Cancer Survival* is the first book to guide you toward transforming your cancer into something manageable. It will provide you with critical answers regarding cancer survival as no other book has before.

I've spent more than 12 years collecting this data and insight in order to share it with you here. *Lifelines* is my compilation of the lessons and tools I used personally to stay alive. In this book, you'll find details regarding the step-by-step approach I developed and used to overcome an advanced and one of the most unusual cancers in the world. You'll learn how to:

1. Find your lifelines, including getting multiple opinions

2. Research your illness and acquire personalized care

3. Discover your own targeted, customized treatment strategies

This guide will show you how to set your intention to survive, build your inner circle, create your "Triad of Survival" (multiple back-up plans), personalize your care, perform critical research, seek multiple opinions, include anticancer nutrition, and get spiritual guidance, as well as financial support.

Futuristic cancer treatment is available now, today. And when you're introduced to what's out there, you may be surprised. Indeed, many of the lifelines you'll read about in these pages are not typically found in conventional medicine. But they're often just as important, if not more important, for you to be aware of. Then, armed with essential information about your options, your real options, you can make the right choices and take the right actions to extend your own life.

How did I arrive at these strategies? It started on a day I'll never forget: December 30, 2002. It was a cold, dark, blustery day outside. I was inside a large teaching hospital where the staff was scurrying to begin the day's work. The first patient they wheeled into the operating room that day was me—a middle-aged man starting the fifth decade of life. I was a hard-working physician's assistant and runner who had collapsed just two days before. I was feverish, had dangerously low blood pressure, and was not stable enough for an anesthetic.

My imaging studies revealed multiple malignant tumors that had spread into all eight quadrants of my liver. Furthermore, the disease was so extensive that it was extending out into my lungs. To save my life, my medical team needed to know my primary diagnosis.

After I was draped, the interventional radiologist inserted a large, thick needle into the side of my abdomen. I grimaced and bore the pain. After 20 minutes of searching and probing, the physician told me they would have to gain entry to my liver by going through my chest. The nurse inserted a tongue depressor into my mouth so I could bite down on it to help me cope with the agony. Then, they inserted a larger needle through my ribs while tidal waves of pain overtook me. During the height of this agony, the tongue depressor split in two.

Forty-eight hours later, the oncologist came into my hospital room to give me the news. "You have cancer all over your liver and lungs," he said. "Not only that, this is one of the rarest sarcomas in the world, and it's unresponsive to all known chemotherapy." I asked, "Doc, how much time do I have?" "Probably three to six months," he replied.

That was 12 years ago.

♥

With this, you have some idea of how my odyssey began. Like every person who faces a deadly diagnosis, I had to choose whether to live or die. I chose to cling to life. Additionally, I had to develop cutting-edge strategies and skill sets to keep myself alive.

In today's healthcare arena, it's mandatory that you do the same in order to survive. *When any of us are hit with cancer, it's what we don't know that can kill us.* This book was written specifically for you and your family to ask the right questions and find the correct answers to keep you around.

Remember, no matter how dire your circumstances, there is always hope. These steps helped me beat the odds, and they can help you, too.

Chapter 1

Lifelines —Tools for Survival

"Two roads diverged in a wood, and I —
I took the one less traveled by,
And that has made all the difference."
— Robert Frost

Each day in the United States, almost 1,600 adults and kids—enough to fill four jumbo jets—die of cancer.[1] Why are these patients allowed to crash and die? We have put people on the moon. We have sent rovers to Mars. Why, in the 21st century, are we throwing up our hands and saying, "There is nothing more we can do"?

Cancer patients need answers and they need them now. *Lifelines to Cancer Survival* bridges the gap from the old world of cancer care to a new, revolutionary way of thinking. What is this new way of thinking, and how is it transforming cancer survival?

It's a way of thinking that empowers you with what I call "lifelines." Lifelines are tools, strategies, and individuals that can help increase your survival time. They can be anything from simple anticancer nutrition, to the latest, cutting-edge genetic profiles and targeted treatments.

---

1. Cancer Facts & Figures, 2014, http://www.cancer.org/acs/groups/content/@research/documents/web-content/acspc-042151.pdf.

The current standard of care can fall short. It often does not include the following individualized tests and treatments that could lead to safer, more effective care:

1. **Personalized molecular profiles**—genetic fingerprints of the potential therapeutic targets of your specific cancer

2. **Anticancer nutrition**—evidence-based natural therapies that attack inflammation and blood vessel growth in your tumor(s)

3. **Integrative medicine**—natural, more holistic modalities to address stress and the side effects of chemo and radiation, along with spirituality

4. **Chemosensitivity assays**—samples of your living tumor or liquid/blood cancer that have been examined and tested to assess your cancer's response to both older and newer anticancer treatments

Your cancer care should include these elements and so much more. My experience in my own survival, and in counseling countless cancer patients over the years, has taught me that staying alive includes much more than a biopsy, chemotherapy, and surgery.

Mark Meets Cancer

I recall my initial introduction to cancer, the "emperor of all maladies,"[2] when I was 21 years old. It was 1976, and I had just completed my Bachelor of Science degree at Central Michigan University. I was working as an orderly in the emergency room at Ingham Medical Center hospital in Lansing, Michigan to gain experience towards a medical degree.

It was Christmas Eve. I was cleaning up a procedure tray in the ER when they wheeled a new patient into the cubicle. Walking back to her station, the triage nurse

---

2. Siddhartha Mukherjee, *The Emperor of All Maladies: The Biography of Cancer*, 2010.

asked me to start taking the woman's medical history. I could see the patient's weary, frightened, blue eyes as I made my way toward her stretcher. She had a lovely, pointed nose and dark-grey hair with white streaks. She told me that she had been diagnosed with late-stage gastrointestinal cancer 12 months earlier and had just finished another round of palliative chemotherapy. Over the past few days, she had been dizzy and had experienced numerous falls. Prepping her for evaluation by the emergency room physician, I took her vital signs and glanced over her pale, thin body. Taking my hand in hers, she confided to me that this would be her last Christmas on this earth, and it made her very sad. She went on to tell me how much she would miss her children and grandchildren when she was gone. Tears streamed down her cheeks, and my heart sank to the floor. This was my first face-to-face experience with an end-stage cancer patient.

Not six months later, I was assigned to care for a 39-year-old man, married with children, who was in the later stages of acute leukemia. I took his vitals, gave him fluids, and changed and turned him to keep him comfortable for my 10-hour shift. He was of average height, his muscles were wasting, he was thin, and his skin was dark-brown as a result of liver failure. I often had to adjust his oxygen mask over his sad, sullen face. He was too weak to talk and he could hardly breathe. There was a quiet, stillness in the room that day. I could feel that his march toward death was nearly over. He had no visitors while I was there. I felt helpless and terribly depressed. Such frustrating and devastating experiences continued as I progressed to physician assistant and an integrative clinician. At the time, I had no idea that 30 years later, I would be the patient on the bed fighting off the horrible, dark disease called cancer.

I have worked hard to forge a way through hell and back to survive. My survival isn't just luck. One of the primary reasons I survived is because I filled in the gaps that I experienced while traveling to numerous oncology offices all over the country. Though some of my oncologists played critical roles in keeping me alive, others were lacking the education, experience, and knowledge in a range of integrative protocols.

These ranged from basic anticancer nutrition to genetics, diet, exercise, supplements, and targeted treatment that certainly contributed to my survival.

In his compelling book, *Anticancer: A New Way of Life,* scientist, physician, and researcher, the late Dr. David Servan-Schreiber discusses his frustration and concerns over this topic as a recovering cancer patient:

> After surgery and chemotherapy for cancer, I asked my oncologist for advice. "What should I do to lead a healthy life, and what precautions could I take to avoid a relapse?" "There is nothing special to do. Lead your life normally. We'll do MRI scans at regular intervals, and if your tumor comes back, we'll detect it early," replied this leading light of modern medicine.
>
> "But aren't there exercises I could do, a diet to follow or to avoid? Shouldn't I be working on my mental outlook?" I asked. My colleague's answer bewildered me. "In this domain, do what you like. It can't do you any harm. But we don't have any scientific evidence that any of these approaches can prevent a relapse." . . . As for more theoretical mind-body or nutritional approaches, he clearly lacked the time or interest to explore these avenues.

Dr. Servan-Schreiber is not alone in this experience. Despite the sometimes dramatic gains made in the treatment of certain types of cancer and leukemia, cancer is now the second leading cause of death in the United States. Second only to heart disease, cancer kills close to 600,000 people a year. In another 16 years, cancer will surpass heart disease and become the leading cause of death in the United States. In fact, the number of new cancer cases is expected to increase nearly 42 percent by 2030, from 1.6 million cases to 2.3 million cases annually.[3]

What's more disturbing is that people will not only die from cancer, but from complications of cancer treatment. Integrative oncology pioneer Dr. Keith Block

---

3. Laura Trent, "The State of Cancer Care in America, 2014: A Report by The American Society of Clinical Oncology," *Journal of Oncology Practice,* http://jop.ascopubs.org/content/10/2/119.full.

says, "While most cancer patients don't die from their disease, they unfortunately and unnecessarily can die from the complications associated with the disease and its related treatments." I agree with his assessment, that taking steps to prevent or mitigate these complications can be a life-saving strategy.

Often, Dr. Block suggests cancer patients may struggle with:

- "Wasting syndrome," known as cachexia

- Infections, with fevers and neutropenia (low neutrophil count, a type of cell that helps make up the white blood cells that fight infection)

- Thromboembolism (blood clots usually starting in the veins of the lower extremities that can travel to the lungs)

- Pain syndrome (intractable pain resulting from cancer or its treatment)

Despite the information promulgated by the American Cancer Society and the National Cancer Institute on lifestyle modifications that can prevent cancer, it is estimated that 1,658,370 new cancer cases will be diagnosed and 589,430 people will die from cancer in the United States in 2015.[4] Based on statistics I have seen, cancer will become the most common cause of death in the U.S. in the net two decades. Many cancer patients do not even realize what they are up against. Some studies suggest that two-thirds or more of cancer patients with a poor prognosis incorrectly believe the treatments they receive could cure them.[5]

Sadly, a significant percentage of people diagnosed with cancer will have shorter lives because they lack the knowledge of potentially lifesaving therapeutic options. And that's what I want to share with you. There are numerous, often untold, lifelines that saved my life.

---

4. American Cancer Society, 2015, http://www.cancer.org/acs/groups/content/@editorial/documents/document/acspc-044552.pdf.

5. Lauran Neergaard, "Report Finds Aging U.S. Faces Crisis in Cancer Care," *Huffington Post*, September 9, 2013, http://www.huffingtonpost.com/2013/09/10/cancer-care_n_3902356.html.

Anything Is Possible

It's evident that there is a wide chasm—even a disconnect—between cancer research and clinical oncology. Groundbreaking discoveries are made regularly, but
most patients and even some oncologists are not aware of them. Moving slower
than a turtle, and sometimes at glacial speed, the progress from research bench to
clinical application for certain tumors is barely discernible. This is frustrating for
millions of cancer patients, like me, who have been diagnosed with rare tumors.
Patients facing these tough cancers, which impose an extremely tight timetable,
need answers now. There are many reasons why these delays are so prevalent, but
they are beyond the scope of this book. Yet it's exactly that concern and frustration
over these gaps in bringing research to clinical application that inspired this book.
Remember this: No matter how frustrating, no matter what the circumstance, no
matter how dire your prognosis, *there is always hope.*

There are thousands of cancer patients who have extended their survival well
beyond the average, or who are seemingly cured after being given a terminal
prognosis. They are called "exceptional" patients. What is it that they are doing
to heal themselves of incurable diseases or to improve their chances of being
cured?

Kelly Turner, PhD, author of *Radical Remission: Surviving Cancer against All Odds*,
has studied more than 1,000 examples of "spontaneous remission," as it is often called.
Typically, there is nothing spontaneous about these unusual cases. Most of these patients are actually doing something to facilitate healing. According to Dr. Turner, there
were nine factors common to most of the patients. These people:

- Radically changed their diets

- Took control of their health

- Followed their intuition

• Used herbs and supplements

• Released suppressed emotions

• Increased positive emotions

• Embraced social support

• Deepened their spiritual connection

• Had strong reasons for living

Moshe Frankel, MD, has also done research on exceptional outcomes and found "connections" to be a common theme. There were internal connections, meaning a relationship with God or a higher power, and with oneself. And there were external connections, or those with family and friends, the medical system (physicians, nurses, and other staff), and other patients. Personal activism was another recurrent theme that involved taking charge, getting engaged in the process of diagnosis and treatment, being more altruistic in one's relationships with others, and changes in philosophy of life.

Toward Safer, More Effective Cancer Care
Crucial lifelines, such as personalized care, may or may not be found in your oncologist's office. But the answer is more complicated. Other critical lifelines you'll read about here, such as personalized vaccines, anticancer nutrition, animal surrogates, and other strategies might very well be found only outside the office. Moreover, of all the available lifelines, only a small percentage of patients are aware of these real opportunities; they often may not realize which precise lifelines could be potentially lifesaving for them. This book focuses on the specific, targeted strategies/therapies of which most patients are unaware.

Lifelines will help you build and maintain a personalized treatment plan, or what I call the *Triad of Survival*. The Triad of Survival is a crucial element of any cancer patient's journey. It is a fluid, constantly updated set of targeted treatment plans developed by you, your oncologist, and your inner circle. More on this critical lifeline is discussed in Chapter 4.

Following your initial diagnosis, you may find an overwhelming amount of material coming from well-meaning doctors, family, and friends. The information you find here will help you discern the *most critical factors* in keeping you alive. Survival encompasses a whole package of things you need to do, even though it is sorely tempting to be a good, "compliant" patient and just take a pill, without doing anything else to help you survive.

Cancer patients with advanced, unusual, or aggressive disease often need to go above and beyond the typical standard of care. They also need to understand the basics of survival, including outside the box thinking and tactics, along with more innovative strategies. The tools and lifelines outlined in this book may very well help you to stick around.

Of the many lifelines I tapped into, below is a short list of my integrative medical lifelines. You can see that it is hard work to stay alive. Clearly, I've had more than one doctor and have used more than one treatment! When people ask, with great trepidation, "Do you think I should get a second opinion," I can't help but smile. Take a look at my history:

- Several leading-edge liver procedures, including a transplant and radio frequency ablation

- 20+ oncologists

- 7 liver surgeons

- 5 interventional radiologists

- Countless medical opinions from medical centers in Michigan, Ohio, Illinois, California, Texas, New York, and Massachusetts

- Numerous phone consults, including those with:
  - Memorial Sloan-Kettering Cancer Center
  - University of Pittsburgh Medical Center
  - Mount Sinai Hospital in New York City
  - Tufts Medical Center
  - University of Massachusetts General Hospital

- Physicians in Europe, including:
  - Germany
  - Great Britain
  - Switzerland
  - Austria

- Countless immune boosting IVs

- 6 different chemotherapies

- 2.5 years of clinical trials

And this is the short list! As you can see, it takes intention, hard work, discipline, and persistence to stay alive when you're diagnosed with a serious cancer.

Dr. Keith Block writes in his book, *Life over Cancer*, "Cancer is not something you want to face alone," and "whom you choose to see you through will affect your quality of life and your chances of attaining and sustaining a full remission." Time after time, I have watched many patients try to go it alone. That is to say, they try fighting an aggressive or late-stage cancer by themselves with the first oncologist to whom they are referred. As the treatment goes on, countless patients run out of options and succumb quickly to their disease, or to the complications or side effects of their treatments. Many are unaware of the numerous risks and potentially limited benefits of treatment options, tests, and procedures. Don't be afraid to look for a researcher or strategist to help you understand your illness. They can also help you navigate a very complicated medical maze.

Regardless of what we are told, the war on cancer is far from being won. There are critical gaps in the standard of care, such as the lack of anticancer nutrition and other cutting-edge tests and treatments. It's my goal to offer you plenty of lifelines to help you close these gaps. Patients facing difficult malignancies, like myself, do not have time to wait. These tools and modalities are already in place. Now is the time to use them.

Summary

I want you to understand that at the present moment, we are walking between two worlds: the traditional, conservative standard of care and a bold, new world of personalized cancer care. We have the knowledge, resources, and technology to fight many types of cancer. What we don't have is a process to know when and how to use them. I know what it's like to be up against the wall with limited or no options for survival. But the multidimensional approach you'll be learning about in these pages has extended my life, and it may help extend yours, too.

> *"You can rise above this.*
> *There is a way through it.*
> *You can survive."*
> — Mark Roby

Chapter 2

Lifelines to
Setting Your Intention to Survive

" . . . The moment one definitely commits oneself, then Providence moves too. All sorts of things occur to help one that would never otherwise have occurred . . . which no man could have dreamed would have come his way. Whatever you can do, or dream you can do, begin it. Boldness has genius, power, and magic in it. Begin it now."
— Johann Wolfgang Von Goethe

The old notion of the all-knowing doctor and the passive, compliant patient still works some of the time. But if you're facing a life-threatening illness, there's a good chance that this outcome may not be optimal. Not because doctors aren't trying, but because cancer is one of the most complex, sly, sophisticated illnesses to ever plague humanity. Its sole purpose is to destroy mankind as it takes your body's nutrients, blood supply, and immunity, and uses it against you. Therefore, it's critical that cancer patients become informed and engaged, and that they set their intention to survive.

If I had not taken the bull by the horns, researched my illness, and been engaged in my care, I wouldn't be alive today. If I had been a "good," compliant patient who only followed the options that were laid out for me, I would be a dead man. What many patients don't ask themselves is What do I have to *do* to stay alive? What do I have to *know* to stay alive? What are the *actions* I need to take right now to stay alive? What kind of *skill sets* do I need to learn to stay alive? And in the end, it comes down to this critical question: Do I deserve to make my survival the most important thing in my life above everything and everyone else?

If you've been diagnosed with any cancer, but especially an unusual, advanced, or aggressive cancer, you've got to find answers to these questions. If you can't find them yourself, you must reach out to others to help you answer these questions. The lifelines in this book will guide you to find the answers.

Here are some of the elements you can use to set your intention to survive:

- **Focus on your survival**—You need to put your recovery first, before anything else. You can't help your loved ones if you are critically ill or worse. Delegate, delegate, delegate.

- **Research**—Learning about your illness is a critical lifeline that many patients do not realize. Being educated about newer treatment options could be a life or death issue.

- **Define rituals**—Find practices and habits that help you structure your day and focus on healing. This develops discipline, which can increase survival times.

- **Select imagery**—Imagine what it would be like to be whole and cancer-free. What would that look like? What would it feel like? Ask yourself, "What are the steps I have to take to learn how to meditate?"

- **Make lists**—Making lists can help you prioritize your tasks and keep you on course.

Defining Intention and Engagement

It's imperative that the cancer patient and his or her inner circle focus much of their attention on creating a battle plan for survival. Over the past three decades, I've witnessed hundreds of patients with good intentions flounder, partly because of a lack of engagement in their own healing, and partly because safer, more targeted options were not available. *Webster's Dictionary* has various synonyms for "intention," such as intent, purpose, aim, end, objective, and goal. It goes on to define a goal as "something attained only by prolonged effort or hardship."

Surviving a diagnosis of a tough, complicated cancer is hard work. It's a daily, step-by-step process. One must focus an enormous amount of time and energy on survival. If you are too sick, or otherwise unable to take an active role in managing your care, then you must find intelligent, devoted, and motivated individuals to bring into your inner circle.

Setting your intention to survive and then taking action will help you save your own life. I cannot emphasize this enough. While intention is the *thought,* engagement is the subsequent *action.* Engagement is as important as intention, because it is the *action* you take that sets your intention into motion. *Both intention and engagement start in the mind. Life and death are held in the power of our thoughts.*

It's hard to truly appreciate this concept. But as early as the 1970s, Dr. David Spiegel's work with patients who had aggressive breast cancer showed a difference in survival rates between engaged and non-engaged patients. Dr. Spiegel's influential 1989 study reported that group therapy helped women with breast cancer cope and live longer.[6]

One of the ways in which you can become an engaged patient is by developing your health literacy. Learn and understand medical terminology related to your condition. Another is to collect copies of all of your medical records, scans, and test results. Construct your own medical chart in a binder, just like doctors did before the

---

6. American Cancer Society, http://www.cancer.org/treatment/treatmentsandsideeffects/complementaryandalternativemedicine/mindbodyandspirit/support-groups-cam.

advent of electronic medical records (EMRs). Sadly, most EMRs are not readily trans-
ferable between medical facilities, so I urge you to create your own "hard copy."

Using tabs and dividers, place your records in chronologic order, labeled:

- Discharge Summaries

- Consultations

- Progress Notes (These can be written by you as a diary, notebook, or summary of events—study them!)

- Imaging (MRIs, CT scans, x-rays, ultrasounds, nuclear scans, echocardio-
grams, etc.)

- Laboratory Tests

- Miscellaneous (e.g., names and contact information for doctors,
hospitals, imaging centers, and health care personnel)

These steps prepare you to go forward with getting multiple opinions, either
in person or through phone consultations. They also can assist you during a phone
consultation, helping you gather additional information and data about the details
of your illness. A significant percentage of patients facing tough cancers do neither
of these steps and pay a very high price. Armed with my notebook, I have met a
number of clinicians via phone who were more than happy to share critical information with me concerning my diagnosis.

Researching Your Cancer

To survive, I knew I would have to research everything I could about this rare
sarcoma. I gathered information from three sources: hospital and medical center
libraries, Internet searches, and my communications with the Internet support

group International Hemangioendothelioma, Epithelioid Hemangioendothelioma and Related Vascular Disorders (HEARD), for my form of cancer.

Every day I compiled data about the nuances of my tumor. Monthly, I posted summaries of what I'd learned and took them with me to my oncology appointments. This information has been invaluable in keeping me alive.

I knew I would have to hit this cancer with everything I had. That meant determining the actions required to launch a full, frontal attack on my sarcoma. I started buying notebooks and putting titles on the covers, such as Anticancer Nutrition and Newest Conventional Therapies.

I know in my heart that my integrative protocols did indeed help me tilt the balance between life and death. Integrative medicine helped address the missing links in standard oncology, such as a compromised immune system, blood vessel growth within the tumor (angiogenesis), muscle wasting (cachexia), inflammation, malnourishment, and weight loss.

The Importance of Following Rituals
Some people think rituals are religious, cultlike, eccentric, or a reflection of an obsessive-compulsive personality, but we all practice rituals, even if we don't call them that. In my case, the series of practices I developed as my morning "ritual" helped me to build my immune system, cleanse my mind and body, and focus my attention on healing. Here is my routine, which you can use as inspiration to create your own:

- Each morning I arise at 6:00 a.m. and drink my whey protein shake with super greens (e.g., wheatgrass, barley greens, kale—super sources of cancer-fighting omega 3 fatty acids, chlorophyll, and glutathione) and take several vitamins and other supplements.

- I get quiet and pray for five to 10 minutes.

- My prayers prepare me for 15 minutes of spiritual reading.

- Finally, I spend 10 to 15 minutes on imagery and meditation.

I still perform these important steps each day. These simple practices get me relaxed and better able to steer my ship through any rough waters ahead. One of my rituals, using imagery, deserves a bit more explanation.

Over the past 30 years of my practicing medicine, countless cancer patients have discussed the benefits and feeling of well-being they received from going through guided imagery exercises. In order to become whole again, I realized imagery would be crucial to my success. Many successful cancer survivors, business men and women, and athletes will tell you the same thing. Practicing these techniques not only leads to lower stress levels, but also disciplines the mind and body towards more positive results. Here's something you can try:

- Lie down or get into a relaxed position to practice these three
  basic concepts.

- Imagine yourself in complete remission: What would you look like?
  What would you be doing? Where you would be traveling?

- Picture yourself performing the steps it would take to get there, i.e.,
  eating a specialized diet, exercising, and researching your own illness.

- Envision yourself going out weekly and helping other people with
  cancer. Yes, helping others is an essential part of your own healing.

The daily practice of purposefully calling up these images while in a relaxed state can help strengthen and bring clarity to both your conscious and unconscious mind. It also can help you to think more positively and feel inner peace.

Another ritual I established early on, during my respite periods, was making lists of critical lifelines. That practice really helped me to prioritize my strategies and stay on course. I made all kinds of lists, including those for:

- Potential members of my survival team

- Cancer centers and professionals who could give me multiple opinions and/or phone consults

- Contingency plans or my "Triad of Survival" (more on this in Chapter 4)

- Data and research about my tumor type

- Different types of targeted therapy based on cancer-specific genes found in my tumor (genomic therapy)

- Different types of integrative medicine targeted for my tumor

- Financial support

In order to engage myself, I did my research and I developed rituals, lists, and imagery to help discipline my thinking, time, and actions in the midst of chaos. These tools helped me to stay on course, reinforce my intentions, and steer me away from the negativity of a toxic prognosis. This approach helped calm me down and clear my thinking so that I could better hear my inner voice.

I started these lists 10 years ago, but I still use them today. Even though they change and I add to them, the practice of making lists and the information in them is still helping me, and others, to survive cancer. These lists also helped me to feel safer. I had done the hard work of building a safety net of knowledge and data related to my sarcoma. Like many cancer patients, my situation changes often, even in remission. Fighting this type of cancer is a lifelong challenge and requires constant vigilance.

Setting Your Intention

The most important question you will ever ask yourself is *What will it take for me to survive?* Determining the answer to this question is the most essential thing you will do. Failing to ask and answer this question could lead to disaster. The doctors can help guide you through this process, but it is your responsibility to be completely engaged. Because of the voids in conventional oncology, it is *your* job to research the nuances of your tumor type. Why? Because today's standard of care often does not include integrative medicine or personalized cancer care. I strongly urge you to make your survival a priority . . . over work and other areas of your life. Nothing is more important than you and your survival!

Although what I shared above may seem obvious, my experience is that many cancer patients do not fully and consciously set their intention to survive, above all else. Typical questions I hear include:

- What about my kids?

- What about my job?

- What about my spouse?

- What about all of my responsibilities?

Patients tell me, "I can't just push everything aside and focus on me. That's unreasonable." They don't realize that you can't split your focus to survive with trying to also be logical, practical, and responsible. Surviving is so difficult in itself that it needs your full attention.

I've seen it happen over and over again. I'm not saying that you should be irresponsible and neglect those other important aspects of your life. I am saying that what you can do is delegate, delegate, and delegate some more. That's why it's imperative upon your initial diagnosis to send out a call for help. You need all the help and support you can get. Now is the time!

There are many conscious and unconscious reasons why we resist setting the intention for our own survival. For one, a diagnosis of cancer brings up a lot of issues about self-worth. Many of us have never learned how to deeply and truly love and accept ourselves, and it's very difficult to learn overnight. Because of a lack of self-worth, many of us subconsciously defeat ourselves. It's a matter of loving yourself enough to save your own life. The essence of your being is love (which is a Principle of Attitudinal Healing). Ask yourself, "Do I deserve to make my survival the most important thing in my life, above everything and everyone else? Can I do that?"

Another reason we avoid setting our survival intention is that many of us have lived our lives in denial concerning many painful issues, therefore, we haven't dealt with them. We just don't have inner conversations with ourselves about things that matter. So when we are hit with cancer, the reality of the seriousness goes underground, like all the other painful, raw issues we haven't dealt with. What helps, in my experience, is praying for the strength to deal with your cancer head on.

A Cancer Diagnosis Offers a Watershed Moment

Cancer is a turning point and calling from above that something is seriously wrong in your life. It's a watershed moment to change many things. Now is the time to wake up. Freely discuss the challenges of change with someone you trust. I know this is difficult for everyone. It's human nature to stay in our comfort zone rather than jump into the unknown. Fear makes us cling to the familiar even more, whether it's our choice of food, people, routines, etc.

Cancer should lead you to examine every aspect of your life. It should lead you to face the very large, pink elephant sitting in your living room, which likely has been there for quite some time. It's our tendency in Western culture to deny any number of issues, shortcomings, and challenges, especially when they feel overwhelming. Thus, many cancer patients avoid unfamiliar contemplation and introspection, and fall continually into fear and panic. Many will do anything to escape or hide from the battle. It happened to me, too. But then God gave me the insight, grace, and strength to create and implement a battle plan.

Focusing your intention on survival means just that. You need to let go of bad habits, foods, thoughts, relationships, and emotions—and start over. You need to think about letting go of smoking, drinking, certain television shows, toxic people, and negativity. You need to "clean out the closets of your life."

Key Points

No one tells patients that they need to take control of their own disease situation. This is not the time to be complacent. Simply following orders is not enough. Here are some of the key points we covered related to becoming engaged and surviving:

- The importance of setting your intention to survive

- How intention leads to engagement

- The notion that no one has more responsibility for fighting this disease than you do

- Why we resist setting the intention to survive

- How a diagnosis of cancer can offer a watershed moment to change

- The importance of avoiding negative and toxic people

Lifelines/Action Steps

Intention and engagement make us feel alive and give us purpose. Taking action, even small steps, will help you create a more positive and hopeful outlook and put you in charge of your care. The following are actions to help you set your intention and become more engaged:

- Write out your intention to survive. Develop your intention into a simple verse that you can repeat internally over and over, such as, "There is a way through this." Speak it out privately and publicly.

- Make lists of your priorities and goals.

- Buy and use a daily planner. Create daily disciplined schedules and structure personal rituals and/or healthy habits (making health shakes, taking regular walks, reading self-help books, doing research, etc.).

- Get and maintain copies of all of your medical records, scans, and test results.

- Research and develop your own healing imagery. There are countless CDs and workshops on the subject of healing imagery produced by cancer patients, hospitals, and health gurus.

- Study the following websites:

  - *http://www.mdanderson.org*—This site offers a great glossary that will help you learn medical terms related to cancer. (You can find it by searching for "cancer glossary" or by going to http://www.mdanderson.org/patient-and-cancer-information/cancer-information/glossary-of-cancer-terms/index.html.

  - *http://www.mylifeline.org*—Find cancer specific resources, post requests for help or donations, and update everyone at once.

  - *http://www.cancer101.org*—Learn about your disease through multi-faceted resources, create a custom toolbox for managing your diagnosis, and partner with your healthcare team.

■ *www.ihadcancer.com*—Explore this private social support network that connects people who have been there with the people who are there right now: survivors, fighters, and support.

■ *http://www.epatientdave.com*—Learn from cancer survivor and author Dave deBronkart how to take control of your care as an engaged patient. Another great resource offered on this site is *Let Patients Help!: A Patient Engagement Handbook*.

■ *www.cancercare.org*—This site offers many resources, including counseling to manage the emotional and practical aspects of cancer care; support groups; workshops in which leading oncology experts provide the latest, in-depth information about cancer; publications; and resources for financial assistance.

Summary

Do you want to risk your life by being a passive, "good" patient, who does *solely* what your doctor tells you and nothing more? Or do you want to be an engaged, informed, empowered patient with multiple strategies and options who survives? These are the *paramount* questions you need to ask yourself. In upcoming chapters, you'll learn about the strategies that are often overlooked.

> *"You can rise above this.*
> *There is a way through it.*
> *You can survive."*
> — Mark Roby

Chapter 3

Lifelines to Building Your Inner Circle

"None of us is as smart as all of us."
— Ken Blanchard

*"It is amazing what can be accomplished
when nobody cares about who gets the credit."*
— Robert Yates

*I*t was a hot summer night last July when I collapsed on the couch after a tough day at work. When I awoke and glanced at the coffee table, a magazine caught my eye. There she was, a female version of me. I couldn't believe it. This woman had a similar, rare, advanced sarcoma and was still undergoing treatment. The article said the woman had lived longer than anyone on record—more than 25 years—after being diagnosed. Initially, the medical authorities gave her a grim prognosis with very little hope of surviving. As a result, the woman decided that she would do anything to live, she would leave no stone unturned.

Keys to Survival
How did she beat the odds? She became engaged in the process, she built her inner circle, she researched her tumor, and she sought out personalized care, which are

the steps or lifelines that I'll teach you in this book. This woman had been deathly ill numerous times, but sought out multiple opinions from experts all over the country. Taking that course of action led to progressive, lifesaving procedures and contingency plans.

Furthermore, she sought out and delegated tasks to her inner circle/survival team. Her husband became her advocate and navigator. He took detailed notes on the phone and during all of her doctor visits. He made a master file of her medical records, labs tests, scans, and consultations. He knew he had to boost his health literacy, so he started reading websites, medical books, and glossaries. He would also troubleshoot and take care of roadblocks and problems as they arose.

She asked her son to assist her in researching her tumor in its microenvironment (meaning the tumor's molecular structure, blood vessel growth, and amount of inflammation). He was a bulldog, as he tirelessly searched the Internet, went to medical libraries, and sought out experts.

Finally, she and her inner circle recruited an integrative medicine specialist to help her attack the tumors on all fronts, especially nutritionally. She knew nutritional therapy was a critical lifeline towards addressing inflammation and immune suppression.

This woman is my role model, my teacher, and my hero. Why? Because she knows that if she wants to stay alive, she needs to become engaged, secure lifelines, and demand personalized care. Another important point here is that even though this woman has a husband and children, she realized she had to make survival her number one priority. By doing so, she has more time and years to give and share with her family and loved ones.

A Warning to All Cancer Patients (especially those diagnosed with rare, advanced, or aggressive malignancies)

Going it alone with your clinician or medical center, without building a strong inner circle/survival team, could be hazardous to your health. Why is this so?

First, you cannot assume your clinician will do specific, in-depth, genetic research on your own tumor. Second, most clinicians will not know your specific tumor's response to any kind of therapy. Chemosensitivity assays and animal surrogates could assist you towards finding those answers. If you don't have the background or energy to research these important issues, I strongly advise you to seek out individuals who can do this for you. A one-size-fits-all approach often fails.

The mission of this chapter is to give you an understanding of what it takes to fight cancer, regardless of the stage or prognosis. While each case is different, all cancer patients need to surround themselves with a group of eclectic individuals who will help them find out everything possible about their tumor and its microenvironment. You need to understand the *risks and the benefits* of every test, procedure, or treatment that is offered to you. To ignore these critical issues is taking a huge risk.

Defining, Finding, and Building Your Inner Circle
Your inner circle is a group of individuals whom you choose to help keep you alive. Ideally, it would consist of you, your oncologist, family and friends, and others who have the expertise that you need to survive cancer. At a minimum, your circle should include you, your oncologist, and someone to help you research your illness. Ideally, your inner circle would also include an integrative medical practitioner and a family member or friend who could help with day-to-day responsibilities, including child care, grocery shopping, and/or taking you to appointments.

When forming your inner circle, you don't want to make the mistake of putting yourself in a subservient position, which a lot of people do. You are in charge here, the leader, the CEO. You are "hiring" people to help you save your life. When you are approaching new clinicians, it's essential that you find those who fit your needs. You don't want to settle out of desperation for the first one that comes along, or for someone who is a highly regarded "expert" with a distant, aloof attitude and a negative outlook. As Anne Frähm and David Frähm, coauthors of the book *A Cancer Battle Plan*, write:

> In the war against cancer, you're the general. It's your body, your health, your money. Everyone else is "hired" help. Their role is to assist you to accomplish your goal of health and healing by lending their specialized expertise to the project.

Remember, you are hiring and collaborating with the members of your team to save your own life. You deserve the best. Don't settle for less!

Building your inner circle is an important, creative process that is probably going to be ongoing and ever-changing over the course of your cancer treatment. What many cancer patients don't realize is that this is a very critical decision-making process. In my case, it was crucial, and it tilted the balance between living and dying.

From the day of my grim diagnosis, I started calling out for help from my hospital bed. I contacted clinicians at Sloan Kettering and the University of Michigan Medical Center. It took me at least six to eight weeks to find my lead researcher, who was on the staff of MD Anderson in Texas. My inner circle has changed a number of times over the last 12 years, depending upon the severity of my illness. Fighting cancer is a fluid, ongoing process that needs to be continually reevaluated and personalized.

I realize many cancer patients are stressed, anxious, and unsure of the next step to take, and they may not want to be a burden on other people. I want you to realize that from the beginning, you must put out multiple calls for help. The consequences of not doing so are grave. There are people all around you, from every walk of life, who are more than willing to help. The next step is finding the right clinician to fit your needs.

Choosing an Oncologist

Most people spend more time and effort shopping for an appliance, computer, or car than they do looking for an oncologist. They often stay with the first oncologist they meet. While they do rely on family and friends, they need to understand that there is another whole world of help available, or what I call a carefully vetted "inner circle."

If a world-renowned cardiac surgeon was diagnosed with an advanced, aggressive cancer, whom would he or she consult for help? Would he go to the oncologist whose office was closest to his home? Would she go to the specialist she saw on TV? It's my guess that the answer would be a resounding "no"! Who would the average person look for if he or she had cancer? What hallmarks or benchmarks would they use in deciding whom to call? From all that I've learned, very few people would know. Furthermore, what most people don't understand is that you might need much more advice and guidance than what you will get from your local medical provider or family member, if you're facing a life-threatening cancer.

It is *imperative* to find an oncologist who is willing to go the extra mile to provide multiple options, rather than simply a death sentence. If you receive a grim, life-threatening or fatal prognosis, and are only offered palliative chemotherapy (end-of-life chemo) with no hope, you need to move on and consult with another doctor. If I would have stayed with the first two or three oncologists I met, I would not be alive or writing this book.

Oncologists are trained physicians who go through formalized residencies in oncology to become board certified. They gather histories, perform physical exams, and order tests such as blood work, CAT scans, and MRIs (imaging) to determine the origin and stage of a cancer. Moreover, they may bring in consultants on a case, i.e., surgeons, gastroenterologists, and radiologists to assess the need for intervention. Most oncologists are conventionally minded, offering only surgery, chemotherapy, and radiation.

Your initial evaluation and meeting with a new oncologist should be seen as an opportunity to assess how well he/she fits your needs from a number of different angles, including medical knowledge, personality, and sense of empathy and compassion. When choosing an oncologist, it is most desirable to find one *who has seen a fair number of patients with your diagnosis. It is especially important to find one who is eclectic and open-minded, which can be difficult.*

Here is a list of my top criteria to consider when choosing the right oncologist for you, even during your first appointment. You want an oncologist who will:

- **Inspire hope**

  It's helpful to have a doctor who encourages you to fight back.

- **Show empathy**

  Your doctor should listen carefully to everything you say and share. He or she should give you the time that you need during appointments and encourage questions.

- **Connect you with other patients**

  Your doctor may be willing to connect you with patients who received a similar diagnosis and experienced positive outcomes.

- **Be willing to research your case**

  They should be open to looking into and communicating the latest, advanced tests and treatments, if doing so would be to your benefit.

- **Think outside the box**

  What else can be done or tried? It can take unconventional thinking to come up with newer targeted options.

- **Not be afraid to admit he or she does not have all the answers**

  No one has all the answers. And especially when it comes to treating tough cancers, you don't need someone to guess, or to hear empty promises.

- **Refer you to other specialists**
  It could be in your best interest to be referred to another specialist. Your doctor should be willing to do that.

- **Honestly discuss the risks versus the benefits of tests, procedures, and treatments**
  Is that new treatment worth the discomfort and risk? You need all the facts to decide.

There are lots of different ways to find the right oncologist to fit your needs. Start by checking your oncologist's credentials and specialty interests to see what he or she knows about your specific cancer. You may find this information in a simple online search. See if he or she has written scientific papers. Look for oncologists associated with new developments on your type of cancer. You can find them in news articles about cutting-edge therapies. Here are some further tips for finding a good oncologist:

- Ask for personal referrals from cancer patients who were treated successfully.

- Visit http://www.usoncology.com/patients. The **U.S. Oncology Network** is one of the largest cancer treatment and research networks in the country. It includes 1,000 cancer specialists and other resources.

- Refer to the *U.S. News & World Report* peer-reviewed list of top docs in oncology: http://health.usnews.com/doctors/location-index/oncologists.

- It's helpful to have a doctor who encourages you to fight back. Go to the **American Society of Clinical Oncology** (ASCO) membership directory at http://www.asco.org/membership-directory and type in your zip code for a listing of doctors in your area.

- Check out the American College of Surgeons site at https://www.facs.org/. There you'll find information to help you understand surgical procedures or locate a surgeon. Women can access a comprehensive breast cancer glossary of terms.

- Refer to doctors listed at http://www.healthgrades.com. You can search by health condition, location, or procedure. This site offers many resources for patients and includes a rating system for doctors, hospitals, and quality of care.

Most cancer patients do not truly understand what they are up against, and that's understandable. If you are diagnosed with an early-stage or common type of cancer, you might be able to stay alive without much research. But if you or a family member are hit with a complex or difficult cancer diagnosis, it's imperative that you and your inner circle find out everything you can about your tumor type or subtype. Why? Because your disease—your tumor—is unlike anyone else's tumor; it is unique and has many distinct targets and genetic fingerprints. Moreover, your tumor's response or resistance to potential therapies may be learned in advance, if you do your homework. That's why it's critical to have your specific tumor examined very carefully, often more carefully than what the current standard of care requires.

Researchers assist you by finding out the secrets and nuances of *your tumor*. Often, they will search the Internet extensively, looking for scientific papers, articles, and case histories of patients with tumors of a similar type. Furthermore, they might search for important tumor markers (often proteins) or diagnostic tests (chemosensitivity assays and molecular profiles) that may help your oncologist assess your tumor's response to potential therapies. They may seek out eclectic experts who have had success treating your specific type of tumor. And they may search for off-label drugs and integrative therapies that have been effective.

A researcher could be anyone from a medical professional or scientist, to a stay-at-home mom. You might be lucky enough to have your family doctor or nurse help you. Perhaps it is a family member or friend. It could be anyone whom you trust who is committed to your survival. Hopefully, it will be someone who is savvy at using the Internet.

The benefits of having a researcher are many. He or she can:

- Arm you with essential information you often won't find in an oncology office or medical center

- Make cancer less scary by breaking down the information for you and turning the big "C" into a little "c" (He or she can help you put the information in this book into practice.)

- Help translate your medical data and personal research into understandable concepts

- Find and contact healthy survivors with your type of cancer, so you can learn from each other

- Locate experts and help set up phone consultations with them, which could be a critical tool toward gleaning leading-edge treatment options

The Benefits of Having an Integrative Specialist

Integrative medicine is the cautious use of nutrition, natural supplements, acupuncture, meditation, and other natural modalities that augment conventional medicine to fight disease. Integrative clinicians can be oncologists, medical doctors (MDs), doctors of osteopathy (DOs), physician assistants (PAs), registered nurses (RNs), nurse practitioners (NPs), or naturopathic doctors (NDs) who specialize in integrative medicine.

Those who practice integrative medicine consider the whole person, including his or her immune system, lifestyle, overall medical conditions, and nutritional intake, along with personality and emotional and psychological needs. A competent integrative clinician looks at the "bigger picture" and personalizes the treatment plan based on a patient's specific needs. Most cancer patients' needs are unusual in that the anxiety, fear, depression, malnutrition, cachexia (weight loss and muscle wasting), and immune deficiencies are sometimes overlooked in the traditional oncology setting.

The following are some important questions to ask when selecting an integrative specialist:

- How many cancer patients does the practitioner see per year?

- How many courses or didactic training programs specific to integrative medicine has the practitioner attended?

- How long has the specialist been practicing integrative medicine?

- Is he or she affiliated with any complementary/integrative associations, organizations, or institutions? If so, which ones?

- Is the practitioner willing to connect you to his or her current or past cancer patients?

- Is the practitioner willing to help research your specific diagnosis?

The field of integrative oncology is embryonic in its development and is still evolving. Thus, even though many hospitals and medical centers have departments for integrative oncology, few offer residency programs in this specialty.

Aside from that, there are a number of complementary/integrative medical societies. Here are some of them:

- ***American Association of Naturopathic Physicians*** (http://www.naturopathic.org/AF_MemberDirectory.asp?version=2)

- ***American Naturopathic Medical Association*** (http://www.integrativeonc.org/)

- ***Society for Integrative Oncology*** (http://www.anam.org)

Here are some links to oncologists who are experts in the field of integrative medicine:

- Donald Abrams, MD, UCSF, Osher Center for Integrative Medicine (http://www.ucsfhealth.org/donald.abrams)

- Keith I. Block, MD, author and renowned integrative oncologist, whose center is located in Skokie, Illinois (http://www.integrativeonc.org/)

- Brian Lawenda, MD, a radiation oncologist, integrative oncologist, and medical acupuncturist based in Las Vegas (includes information about the AntiCancerize Me Program™ at http://www.integrativeoncology-essentials.com/about/brian-lawenda/)

- Barry Boyd, MD, founder of the integrative medicine program at Greenwich Hospital-Yale Health Systems and author (http://www.drbarryboyd.com)

Finding and Working with Cancer Survivors/Mentors

Cancer survivors are one of the most undervalued and underappreciated sources of wisdom, knowledge, guidance, and inspiration on the planet! Many patients I see forget to tap into this valuable resource. What they may not understand is that the experiences of survivors, gleaned from months or years on the battlefront, could be critical for their survival. Other cancer patients with your specific diagnosis can teach you about the nuances of your condition, the mistakes they've made or witnessed, and cutting-edge information regarding your diagnosis.

Many patients with your diagnosis are often easily accessed either through the Internet or by phone, more so than many medical practitioners who often require that you schedule appointments weeks or months in advance. Also, other patients are often more open and honest about the quality of their care, and/or the efficacy, risks, and benefits of various treatments. They will give you intimate details about the side effects and their feelings associated with certain treatments, or their experiences with specific practitioners, and/or about medical centers that you simply won't get in a medical center or oncology office. They can also be the source of information on unusual or novel therapies that are not part of the standard of care. Moreover, these individuals often give enormous psychological and emotional support to other patients, as they did for me. The importance of this support cannot be understated.

There are thousands and thousands of cancer blogs on the Internet. Look for those with your specific diagnosis, and then vet them by reading what's written. You can also ask your oncologist or specialists for referrals to other cancer patients who were treated effectively. Many survivors have written books, such as Tami Boehmer's *From Incurable to Incredible*. It's basically a compilation of cancer survivors' stories and how they are helping others. Not only is this a great way to find others with your kind of cancer, it gives you an opportunity to vet them based on their writing. Here are some additional ways to find cancer survivors:

- Cancer support groups, in person and online

- Cancer survivor websites (for your particular type of cancer, for example, **www.smartcancerproject.com**)

- Medical centers

- Magazines and publications, such as ***Cure*** and ***Cancer Today***

Use your network and let them know you are looking for other survivors. Unbeknownst to many cancer patients, there is a plethora of ways to find and connect with others facing your diagnosis.

Leaning on Your Family and Friends

Patients often forget when they walk into a medical center that they themselves are the director and CEO of their healthcare. Furthermore, there are numerous articles in the media discussing the dangers and pitfalls of leaning on nonmedical professionals for help and guidance. I think this is nonsense. Why? Because your family, friends, and fellow cancer patients are a critical lifeline to your survival . . . that certainly was true for me. Common sense dictates that empowered, engaged patients, who surround themselves with a myriad of lifelines, will have better survival outcomes than those who don't.

I could not have survived without the love, support, and guidance of my life partner Kathleen. I could never repay her for all she has done for me. In addition, other important members of my inner circle have been my many colleagues and friends. I am deeply grateful for their friendship and support.

Likewise, allow your family and friends to help you. They can act as your scribe during office visits, as well as your researcher, advocate, caretaker, coach, and champion. (Go, baby!) When you are bombarded with an avalanche of information and your emotions are running wild, two heads are better than one. Furthermore, they may offer resources, options, and treatment strategies that your medical team might not even be aware of. If I had not had an army of support, I'm not sure I would be alive today. Cancer is bigger than any one person!

Key Points

Though you are the director of your life, you won't get far without a strong, devoted crew. Now is not the time to go it alone, following the stoic and silent model. At minimum, you will need to "fill" the following positions: oncologist, strategist/researcher, integrative specialist, cancer survivors, and selected friends and family. Your inner circle will help you to fill in the gaps in conventional medicine. In addition, these individuals will help you build contingency plans (I call that the "Triad of Survival," which will be discussed in an upcoming chapter).

Lifelines/Action Steps

Building a strong inner circle should not be taken lightly. It can make the difference between life and death. The sooner you start to search for and assemble your team, the better. Here are some tips to help get you started:

- Do your research using the tools in this chapter to find the best cancer centers and oncologists to meet your specific needs.

- Investigate oncologists and medical centers before seeking care.
  Talk to the staff and ask if you can also talk to patients who have a similar diagnosis. The effort to do this is worthwhile. You'll find an amazing amount of information.

- See certified cancer coach, and a breast cancer survivor, Elyn Jacobs. She empowers women to successfully navigate the process of treatment and care. She's the executive director of the **Emerald Heart Cancer Foundation** and a radio host. Her site offers many resources, including a comprehensive list of integrative medicine specialists (http://elynjacobs.com/).

- See breast cancer survivor and author Tami Boehmer. Her book and website, **Miracle Survivors** (http://www.tamiboehmer.com/), offer inspiration and hope to large numbers of cancer patients on a daily basis. Her compelling story, along with her book, teaches survivors and guides them in how to mentor each other.

- Do your research and find the best oncologist and/or medical center to meet your specific needs.

- If you have an advanced, rare, or aggressive type of tumor, you need to do your homework. This means finding clinical trials with your tumor type and connecting with them. You or your family doctor can have a phone consultation with the staff members who are running the trial. Clinical trial investigators often have more knowledge and expertise regarding your type of tumor than most clinicians. If they are not immediately available for help, ask if they could guide you to an expert clinician in your state.

- Call friends, colleagues, and family, and ask them to assist you in tracking and following through with all of your various appointments. Ask them to accompany you to appointments, take notes, and give you encouragement.

- Delegate critical tasks to family and friends, such as childcare, transportation of kids, meal preparation, laundry, and driving you to appointments.

- The **National Association of Professional Cancer Coaches** offers vital information you won't find elsewhere. Coaches can research your specific tumor and fill in the crucial gaps that are sometimes missing in the standard of care (http://cancerwipeout.org/about.html).

Taking these actions to help build your inner circle will give you a sense of accomplishment and safety. It will also aid in your survival.

Summary

You would be amazed to see and feel the miracles that can come about when you build a strong team. I would not be alive today had it not been for the love, support, and guidance of my inner circle. I have seen countless cancer patients spiral down because they did not understand this critical concept early on. Finding an excellent oncologist, researcher, integrative practitioner, and mentor, along with the support of family and friends, can make all the difference. Your team can provide you with essential knowledge and guidance, as well as inspiration and hope . . . the most important medicine of all. The process of building your team may also lead to you finding multiple opinions, the topic of the next chapter.

"You can rise above this.
There is a way through it.
You can survive."
— Mark Roby

Chapter 4

Lifelines to Your Triad of Survival

"Some authorities think that we cannot solve the cancer problem until we have made a great, basic, unexpected discovery, perhaps in some apparently unrelated field. I disagree. I think we know enough to go ahead now and make a frontal attack with all our forces."

— Dr. Cornelius Rhoads,

1949 archives of *Time*, cover article "Cancer Pioneer"

*T*ruth be told, I had had several premonitions in dreams of my impending doom. In each dream, an entity visited me and kept telling me things like "Why aren't you going to see a doctor? I'm putting this pain in your side and giving you these night sweats for a reason. Take notice! There is something deadly wrong!" In the dream, I asked that if I was going to be sick, it be something I could fight. Upon waking, I felt guilty for neglecting my health and not doing something about my symptoms. That thought nagged at me for months, as I worked harder and ran faster and longer. Little did I know that my worst nightmare was about to come true in the weeks to follow.

The day my life changed forever started routinely. I had showered and then went to the medical center to start a 10-hour stint in the emergency room. Around seven o'clock that evening, I arrived home and started my nightly four-mile run. I can remember it like it was yesterday. The early winter temperature was around 25 degrees and snow had started to fall. I had worked 10 days straight and was so looking forward to these periods of solitude.

I recall that the discomfort I had been feeling in my right abdomen started up again during this run. When I returned home, my whole world started crumbling down around me as I opened the door of my condominium. I had difficulty breathing and felt an excruciating pain in my right ribs as I collapsed. As I lie on the floor, the pain came in waves. Even though I didn't realize it at the time, I had lost 15 pounds and had a fever of 102 degrees. Somehow, I made it to my car and drove to a local trauma center, a large medical facility. The staff thought I might have an acute abdominal issue that would require exploratory surgery. So all they could do in the emergency room was give me intravenous fluids and oxygen. I could have nothing by mouth, and they said it would be dangerous to address the pain without more information. It was one of the most horrific nights of my life.

The next morning, after a battery of tests, I called my father and asked him to be at my side. While he was standing next to me in the emergency room, the attending physician walked in and said he had some bad news. The tests showed I had cancer all over my liver. Not only that, the lesions seemed to be in most of my liver quadrants, and the cancer had metastasized throughout my lungs. They were going to keep me in the hospital to find out the primary source.

Tears started rolling down my face as my father held me. We were both speechless. Here I was, a health nut and a semivegetarian, looking death straight in the eye at 50 years old. Anyone who is initially diagnosed with cancer all through their liver is in big trouble. I was told that I would be facing enormous odds.

Looking for Hope

During the following weeks I visited five hospitals, which included some of the top cancer centers in the U.S., and I had a phone consult with Sloan-Kettering. Each time I hoped to get some good news, some hope. To support my body during this research, I consulted with an integrative physician, who offered me treatments to build my immune system, including intravenous vitamin C, glutathione, and other supplements.

I still remember standing next to the transplant surgeon in the examination room at a major medical center, looking at all of my scans and tests. After about 20 minutes of examining these pictures, he looked at me and said, "Your disease is so extensive throughout your liver and lungs, there is no way we can offer you a transplant. I'm sorry."

The next visit was to a prestigious major cancer center in the Midwest. My fiancée and my family accompanied me. This facility is a teaching hospital, so the doctor who examined me was speaking to a resident oncologist, instructing her about my disease. I overheard him say to her that he thought the disease was in my lungs and bones, and that the prognosis was grim. He suggested the highest level of interferon chemotherapy as a palliative measure.

He gave me a prognosis of roughly 12 to 18 months of life remaining, and told my family the same when he spoke to them in private. He also said I would not be a candidate for a liver transplant. In addition, he stated that besides a liver transplant, there was no known chemotherapy that would stave off or stop my kind of tumor (epithelioid hemangioendothelioma). I felt terribly discouraged and scared about my prognosis. I told him the morphine I was on for pain left me feeling lethargic and in a dream state, and I asked him to put me on a drug called Ultram®, a mild pain reliever that wouldn't dope me up. He wasn't familiar with Ultram® and neither was the resident, so he curtly refused to prescribe it and said I could take either Motrin® or morphine.

I indicated I would go for second and third opinions. The doctor replied, "You're welcome to get those opinions, but I'm sure they're going to tell you the exact same things I did." ***This turned out to be the furthest thing from the truth.*** If I had listened to him and followed the advice of the first four or five cancer centers I visited, I would not be alive today.

For example, I learned from other oncologists that the type of sarcoma I had is often slow-growing, but may change, so I had much more time than he had told me. And there were a myriad of treatment options that he wasn't aware of. In reality, these options, in-cluding a liver transplant, greatly benefitted me and increased my survival time.

My trip to MD Anderson should have been a five-day visit for a consult and treat-ment plan. Instead, they lost my medical records, kept me for four and a half weeks, and as I burned through a hefty chunk of my life savings, they said I was a difficult pa-tient because I complained. In the end, they offered me no hope, only the same palliative chemotherapy that was suggested at the teaching hospitals in the Midwest.

Out of all this hell, stress, and turmoil, I did get one of the most important lessons that helped in my survival, though it did not come from the hospital—it came from a researcher who worked at the hospital. At the advice of my friend, Sherry, I contacted the researcher and he invited me to visit him at his home office. There, he gave me an important survival tool: the concept of having three contingency plans on the table at all times. The work of coming up with these plans has played a major role in saving my life, and I highly recommend you do the same. I call this the "Triad of Survival."

The Importance of a Triad of Survival
The Triad of Survival is one of the most critical elements of any cancer patient's survival. It is an ongoing, updated set of three treatment strategies that are contingency plans. These plans may each be conventional oncology therapies, integrative modalities, or alternative strategies. One can view them as plans A, B, and C. When your current plan fails, you im-mediately choose plan A, B, or C, whichever fits, as your next option. Then, another plan, plan D, must be developed in order to maintain three potential treatment plans waiting in the wings. These plans may also be shuffled in response to new medical challenges. We'll discuss this in more detail in another chapter.

Cancer patients need answers and need them quickly. Our empirically based, clinical trial-driven conventional care works some of the time in early and middle-stage cancers, but nearly 600,000 U.S. adults and children go down each year because of the lack of three basic strategies: 1.) a thorough understanding and surveillance of the enemy; 2.) deception; and 3.) multiple contingency plans. Many medical centers and clinicians ignore or forget these three concepts when treating their cancer patients.

Furthermore, a large majority of patients are not offered advanced/progressive research on their tumors, such as molecular profiles, chemosensitivity assays, animal surrogates, or vaccines. These options could potentially lead to safer, more targeted therapeutic agents. How do I know this? Because I am on such an agent, along with many of my fellow survivors who have done similar research. A number of them are referenced in this book. In war, good commanders plan ahead of time for crisis situations and can fluidly and quickly switch from one strategy to another, depending on the circumstances. Moreover, they already have multiple contingency plans in place well before trouble arises. To beat an intelligent, ruthless opponent like cancer requires an eclectic, flexible approach on multiple fronts, just like history's most successful battles.

Initially you, your oncologist, and your researcher are the most important allies. If you're too sick or too stressed to take the lead role in creating your Triad of Survival, make sure you have intelligent, eclectic, and assertive individuals in your inner circle to assist you. Your inner circle—researching your illness and finding suitable, personalized care options—will help you build your Triad. They can compile the data and work with you to complete your Triad.

The Internet and phone consults are critical lifelines and tools that you can plug into. The more you use these tools, the sooner you will find out how valuable they are. If I had not used these lifelines week by week and month to month, I would not be alive today. They opened up a plethora of knowledge and data that I never thought would be available.

What's Stopping You from Taking Charge?
The question is, How badly do you want to survive? And do you want to leave your fate up to the first oncologist you meet, who might have limited personalized data to draw upon for your care? Many local oncologists may be able to rescue you from an early stage or uncomplicated malignancy, but if you are facing more than that, you might need more eclectic, open-minded professionals to save your life.

One exciting, progressive tool for creating personalized cancer treatments is using mice in place of humans to test the safety and efficacy of older and newer chemo agents. Here's how it works. A sample of your own tumor is removed and then implanted within immunocompromised mice for testing. The goal is to test drugs and treatments on mice before the risky, potentially toxic, life-threatening therapy is used on you.

According to Ronnie Morris, MD, president of Champions Oncology and founder of MDVIP, a national leader in personalized healthcare with a network of 400 doctors, "there is a greater than 80 percent positive predictive value of the treatment working in the patient" when such a protocol is followed. He also says it helps identify treatments that will not have any benefit, sparing the patient from possible toxic side effects.[7]

I asked him whether the current standard of care is enough, if an individual receives a diagnosis of cancer. His response:

> After firstline treatment fails, for most cancers there is only a 10 percent chance of finding an effective treatment option. The process of finding this treatment relies on ineffective population statistics and trial and error, which also takes precious time and exposes patients to toxic side effects of a treatment without benefit. Patients are unable to test multiple treatments at the same time on their own, which is why TumorGrafts are excellent surrogate options. Creating a mouse avatar means that a surrogate tester can be used. That enables identification of a treatment that will likely work, quickly and without harm to the patient.

10 Tools to Build Your Triad of Survival

Below are some valuable tools to help connect you to individuals and resources that will help you build your Triad. Of course, not everything on the Internet is equally useful to cancer patients. These websites use leading-edge technologies that enable you to exchange information about the pros and cons of various treatments, includ-

7. Ronnie Morris, MD, interview with Mark Roby, 2014.

ing side effects, the nuances of tumor types, and personal medical data with other cancer patients around the world:

1   *Champions Oncology*—Another organization that works with your oncologist to find the most targeted treatment available for your tumor. This process takes three steps: implantation (a sample of your tumor is removed and implanted into immunocompromised mice), growth (time is given for the sample tumor to grow in the mice, which can take two months or longer, and you continue to receive treatments during this time), and testing (this organization works with your oncologist to determine which drugs to test on the mice to predict how well they will work for you). You can learn more at http://www.championsoncology.com/.

2   *Smart Patients*—An online community where patients and caregivers learn from each other about treatments, clinical trials, the latest science, and how it all fits into the context of their experience. Find it at http://www.smartpatients.com/.

3   *CureTogether*—Get access to millions of ratings comparing the real world performance of treatments across 637 health conditions. Go to http://curetogether.com/ to learn more.

4   *PatientsLikeMe*—An online community where you can connect with others, gain knowledge about your illness, chart your health over time, and contribute to research. Visit http://www.patientslikeme.com/ for details.

5   *CancerConnect*—Another online community where you meet with other cancer patients, find cancer survival tips, and learn about breaking news. For further information, go to http://news.cancerconnect.com/.

6   *ecancerpatient*—A not-for-profit website that gives cancer patients access to the same information that is currently available to cancer professionals. To get more details, see http://ecancerpatient.org/.

7 ***Providence Health & Services/NantHealth***—For more targeted cancer treatment, Providence Health & Services can connect you to the latest information and technology via NantHealth (http://www2.providence.org/myomics/Pages/default.aspx), a subsidiary of NantWorks. NantWorks was founded by Dr. Patrick Soon-Shiong, who has published over 100 scientific papers, has over 95 issued patents, and is now pioneering genomic sequencing. Providence will be the first healthcare system to use the sequencing system, which will, according to the website, "give the most comprehensive view of each patient's disease available to date."

8 ***PatientCrossroads***—Anyone with cancer can contribute data to this organization and anyone who needs the data can access it. Find out how patients around the world are receiving treatment, vet patient communities for research studies, and get the information you need to make smarter decisions. Learn more at http://patientcrossroads.com/.

9 ***Gradalis®, Inc.***—A late-stage biopharmaceutical company, Gradalis® (http://www.gradalisinc.com/) is focusing on developing novel, personalized therapies to treat cancer. Its proprietary immunotherapy platform, Vigil™, can be used for multiple advanced cancers as long as a sample of the solid tumor can be removed surgically. The goal is to activate the patient's immune system to attack the tumor cells.

10 ***Resource List***—A list of over 50 websites for decision-making, education, information and treatment management, lifestyle management, and social support. Find out more at http://ehidc.org/resource-center/directories/hit-cancer-resource-guide.

These resources, along with your own extended research, will go a long way to help you build your Triad of Survival.

MARGARET CASTEEL

Here is an excerpt from a story written by one of my patients, Margaret Casteel. She is a 61-year-old woman who started feeling ill around Thanksgiving 2013. Two weeks later, she felt worse and became jaundiced. Tests showed her bile duct was completely blocked. Subsequent surgery revealed a malignant, inoperable tumor with protrusions around her gallbladder and liver. She describes waking up after her operation . . .

Margaret's Story

Over the next couple days, my life changed forever. My doctors explained that I had a high-grade, fast-growing, unusual cancer (cholangiocarcinoma, which is bile duct cancer). My options were to either do nothing and die in three or four months, or to try chemotherapy. The prognosis was grim.

My son, Nick, is an avid reader. He researched options and found one medical professional who was a cancer survivor and integrative clinician, Mark Roby, PA-C, who he met through a cancer lecture where Mark had been speaking. Nick took my husband and me to see him at his office. Mark was instrumental at helping all of us stay focused on staying alive. He explained his lifelines concept and tied it into each aspect of my survival. He explained each step, starting with building my inner circle, accessing multiple opinions, researching my tumor, and building my Triad of Survival.

Building my inner circle was easy because I have so many people who helped to point me in the right direction. The inner circle is the group of people who know my treatments, condition, options, and results inside and out. They do the research with me and on my behalf. These are the people I talk with about what my next steps are.

Getting multiple opinions is important because I have an unusual cancer. My doctor had seen less than six cases in total, so why not find out what other options might be out there? Another opinion might even save my life.

The Triad of Survival is about having backup plans in place. Mark suggests people have three options of possible treatments that might work, if the current treatment regimen does not work. He and my son did a ton of research on my condition and various, potential treatments. I feel much safer knowing my Triad is in place.

Many times Nick would do research and then consult with Mark before making a recommendation. My cancer is unusual, and I am in a unique situation. So together, our research showed what I should do to better my odds. I am attacking this cancer from every way I can: I destress, pray, use imagery, relax, exercise daily, take vitamins, have a specialized diet, and include conventional medicine.

Mark suggested that we send the tumor out for a molecular profile, looking for biomarkers. He helped my son find a clinical trial at Cleveland Clinic. They sent samples of my tumor to Foundation One, where they found a genetic target that might be driving my tumor. Currently, we are looking for a clinical trial or other modalities to address this. Mark also told my son about photodynamic therapy (PDT), which Nick has researched extensively.

During the last three to four months, I have had chemotherapy and radiation, which have knocked my tumor markers down and actually shrunk my tumor. We are hoping for more shrinkage and possible removal of the tumor. I am alive and very grateful.

Creating My Own Triad of Survival

Being a medical professional, I thought I had exhausted all of my channels. I felt like a fish out of water, because it seemed like all the medical professionals I had seen were just going to give me palliative treatments. No one except that researcher had given me anything to hold on to. Even some of my friends were encouraging me to accept what the doctors were telling me and to prepare for what they considered to be the "inevitable." But having that Triad of Survival strategy gave me a glimmer of hope. It was something I could *do* and hold on to; it gave me a purpose.

As I stated before, I was on huge doses of interferon that landed me in the hospital. Not only did it make me sicker, it made me seriously ill. It was the summer of 2003 when I just started to awaken from my interferon-induced stupor. It was around that time that I met an oncologist who seemed to want to help me survive. One of the tumor markers on my pathology report was positive for a protein called c-kit. This genetic abnormality was prevalent in my tumor type, and he wanted to start me on a drug called Gleevec® that targeted the c-kit abnormality.

In my free time, I decided to take the advice of my researcher/strategist from Houston and build my first Triad of Survival. I needed to come up with three contingency plans to keep on the table and ready to go at any time.

Let me illustrate how the Triad of Survival works, so that you, in turn, can apply it. The first part of the equation, after the interferon failed, would be starting the Gleevec® chemo in August. Many sarcomas are chemo resistant, but we both thought it was worth a try. If that plan failed (which it eventually did), I would move on to my next option, which would be traveling out west to the Orange County Immune Institute and spend four weeks implementing natural and integrative therapies, such as intravenous vitamin C and glutathione.

The more that I researched my tumor type, the more I realized the need for me to address the vascular aspects of my malignancy. I researched angiogenesis (growth of new vessels inside a tumor) at length and called Dr. Juda Folkman's lab (the "father" of angiogenesis) in Boston. They performed some tests on my urine and sent me the results.

At the same time, I made a list of the foods and supplements that would stop angiogenesis and started to integrate them into my daily protocols. I strongly believe in Dr. Folkman's work and discussed it with my oncologist in Traverse City, Michigan. He agreed to add Avastin® (a drug that stops angiogenesis) as a conventional therapy, and it became part of my third contingency plan, if needed.

Thus, my first Triad of Survival was completed: Gleevec®, the Orange County Immune Institute, and the targeted agent Avastin®. I knew that besides implementing my Triad, it was imperative that I held fast to my strict daily regimens, including prayer, meditation, imagery, exercise, an alkaline diet, and supplements that addressed inflammation. The results of my initial Triad were as follows: The Gleevec® didn't work to slow down or stabilize my tumors, yet my time at the Immune Institute was informative and encouraging, as it did slow down the progression of the tumors but did not completely stop the growth.

In late fall 2004, I started on Avastin®, which stabilized the tumors. However, as time went on, my insurance stopped covering the Avastin® and I had to reassess. Up against the wall, I realized I had to search, study, and search some more. I encourage you to do the same, because there are many roadblocks and mountains ahead that you're going to meet. That's why building and rebuilding your Triad of Survival is critical. When this first Triad lost its effectiveness, I moved on to my next Triad. I tried Ukrain, a non-FDA approved, European chemo; IV alpha lipoic acid; and a new, targeted agent called Sutent®.

Remember, as solutions begin to lose effectiveness, you need to look for new ones so you will always have three in your arsenal. This is what it means to continually build and rebuild your Triad of Survival. This new paradigm keeps you engaged, alive, and gives you peace of mind.

Locating the Best Treatment Options for Your Triad

Could studying the genetic makeup of your tumor help you build a safer, more effective Triad for yourself? The answer is not black and white. But I can say from personal experience that genetic/molecular profiling could possibly offer you more clinical options than the current standard of care. In Dr. Ralph Moss's book, *Customized Cancer Treatment,* Dr. Patrick Hwu from MD Anderson states, "It is an important goal to determine optimal chemotherapy combinations for individual patients to enhance patient response, avoid toxicities, and gain insights that lead to improved treatment strategies."

One critical tool in finding optimum cancer treatment is a molecular or genetic profile of your tumor, which is described more in-depth in the chapter on research. This is often a genetic study of your tumor following a biopsy or surgery. The pathologist sends your physician a report, which would then include a clinically relevant target or targets that may be pursued.

The second essential ingredient would be finding an oncologist who believes in or is well versed in these technologies or personalized care. One such individual is Sandeep Reddy, MD. Board certified in medical oncology and internal medicine, he is chief of staff at Los Alamitos Medical Center in Los Alamitos, California. He also serves as a clinical professor of medicine at the David Geffen School of Medicine at the University of California in Los Angeles (UCLA).

The following is an excerpt of an interview I had with him in fall 2014, where he discussed how molecular profiling may lead to different treatment options.

Mark Roby: Discuss what the current standard of care is and how it is transitioning into the personalized care arena.

Dr. Sandeep Reddy: Currently, standard of care (SOC) is established through randomized clinical trials. These trials test one treatment option versus another and patients are randomized to receive one option. Randomization is done to exclude bias and increase the likelihood that the results will be able to be reproduced in other patients. We are now moving towards a personalized medicine approach that centers on the idea that each patient is a unique individual with his or her own unique cancer. There are biologic features that can be assessed and used to design the most appropriate treatment regimen for that patient; one size does not fit all.

Mark Roby: Briefly explain molecular profiling and its importance in the clinical setting.

Dr. Sandeep Reddy: Every cancer is different in the same way that each of us is different. Our genetic makeups cause each individual to react differently to the same treatments. This makes diagnosing and determining which treatment will work best for that individual's tumor type very challenging. Molecular profiling has achieved this difficult task. Profiling each individual tumor will allow oncologists to assess the tumor's molecular profile and determine what mutations have occurred, allowing them to recommend the most effective treatment.

Mark Roby: Discuss the tumor microenvironment and its influence on patient outcomes, along with tumor growth.

Dr. Sandeep Reddy: The tumor microenvironment, while still a mystery, is becoming better understood. This is leading to new therapies. The understanding of angiogenesis (growth of new blood vessels) has spurred the development of bevacizumab and other agents that target vascular endothelial growth factor (VEGF). When added to chemotherapy, bevacizumab adds 10 percent to the response rate across multiple tumor types. A postulated mechanism of this drug is that bevacizumab binds to VEGF, decreasing new capillary growth, effectively starving the tumor of oxygen and nutrients, also decreasing hydrostatic pressure around the tumor, and thus allowing for greater chemotherapy penetration to the tumor core.

Mark Roby: Could you comment on the current status of targeted therapies and how they differ from the older, traditional chemotherapies?

Dr. Sandeep Reddy: Chemotherapy can be loosely defined as poison. These drugs interfere with vital cellular metabolic processes to kill the cell but are not discriminating in their choice of which cells are affected. Targeted therapies are designed to interact with a specific cellular target, such as surface receptor protein . . . or an intracellular protein . . . Since the drugs only interact with the cellular target, they are highly specific to which cells are affected and, thus, there is usually less toxicity than with conventional chemotherapy. These drugs can be used on their own, or sometimes combined together or with chemotherapy to improve outcomes.

Mark Roby: Could you give some advice or guidance to these points for those who want more effective personalized approaches?

Dr. Sandeep Reddy: Patients must be their own advocates. When fighting a deadly disease, without a high probability of cure with standard therapy, it is very reasonable to "think outside of the box." We live in the era of Google, and so it is the duty of the patient to seek out answers, not just for themselves, but also future patients. Often patients may be dissuaded from trying something new, but as long as these approaches are being tried in the right context (when SOC had failed) and under the proper conditions (physician oversight, a well conducted clinical trial), it is actually the best option for patients.

Key Points

Building your Triad of Survival can make a difference. Month by month, year by year, we all watch as our family members and friends are stolen away by this horrific, ruthless killer. It's imperative that cancer patients *and* their healthcare team use everything at their disposal to win this battle.

- Work with your inner circle to create and research your Triad of Survival.

- Use the resources and websites in this chapter to build your strategies.

- Don't forget to think outside the box.

- It's important to always look ahead and constantly reassess your strategies.

Lifelines/Action Steps

Slowly and methodically, you can and will find ways to save your own life. You can do it. Remember the phrase I wrote in the beginning: *There is a way through it. You can survive.* In the face of numerous death sentences, I would not have survived without my multiple Triads of Survival. Here are some steps you can take:

- Study the websites in this chapter, along with Chapters 6, 7, and 8 to find out everything you can about your tumor and potential treatments.

- Carefully study the risks and benefits of every option you are given.

- Make a master binder or folder with all of your consults, labs, scan results, treatments, and records. Always keep one master at home and a spare for travel.

- Call other cancer patients with your type of tumor and pick their brains as to the benefits and pitfalls of their experiences. These stories could be invaluable.

- Perform Internet searches to assess cutting-edge strategies and clinical trials, then call the principle investigators or authors of the research papers and ask them for information or guidance.

- Work with your inner circle and oncologist to develop and constantly update your Triad of Survival.

- Get away from the drama by yourself and ask God or whatever higher power you refer to for guidance on these issues. Don't give your power away or make major decisions on the spot or out of fear.

Summary

The Triad of Survival is a critical lifeline for patients diagnosed with advanced, aggressive, or rare tumor types. This ongoing, three-step contingency process, consisting of a plan A, B, and C, is essential if you are serious about staying alive.

There are three reasons why having a Triad of Survival is absolutely necessary. First, often your oncologist may not understand the genetic fingerprint of your tumor or your tumor's response to random therapies. Second, the standard of care often does not work. And third, instead of being trapped, the Triad of Survival always gives you multiple strategies of attack and hope.

So work with your inner circle and oncologist to come up with your Triad of Survival. When one of your backup plans gets used up or is proven ineffective, always replace it as soon as you can.

> *"You can rise above this.*
> *There is a way through it.*
> *You can survive."*
> — Mark Roby

Chapter 5

Lifelines to Anticancer Nutrition

"In 1982, the National Research Council released a technical report,
'Diet, Nutrition and Cancer,' showing that diet was probably
the greatest single factor in the epidemic of cancer."
— Neal Barnard, MD, from *Foods Can Save Your Life*

*I*n January of 2003, I had just left the hospital and gone back to my condo in Southeast Michigan. Over a span of eight to 12 weeks (while on chemo), I became weak, malnourished, and exhausted. My weight plummeted from 180 pounds to 140 pounds, and I was becoming progressively emaciated. When I looked at myself in the mirror, what I saw frightened the hell out me. I appeared so pale and skinny, I thought I was about ready to die. Over the next six to eight months, I was put on one chemotherapy drug after another, each one failing to stem the tide. Furthermore, I experienced complicated, dangerous side effects, which often landed me in the hospital. And my weight plummeted further.

When I asked my various Midwest oncologists about these issues, they advised me to eat foods to put on weight, such as hamburgers, steaks, milkshakes, and dairy products. They also suggested a pharmaceutical supplement drink filled with sugar and additives. Apparently, they thought these foods would help with my muscle and weight loss. In addition, they warned me against going on plant-rich diets or taking natural supplements, telling me they were dangerous and would escalate my demise. Yet nothing was further from the truth.

While I was seeking multiple opinions from around the country and receiving my chemotherapy, often the staff members would offer me what I called "gift baskets." They would contain milk chocolate bars, soda, brownies, cookies, and highly refined carbohydrates, such as salted peanuts, crackers, and other junk food. They were well intentioned in their offerings, but what they didn't and still don't realize is that they were throwing fuel on the fire.

The Missing Link

Hypocrates once said, "Let food be thy medicine." Following your diagnosis, each morsel of food you consume is just as important as surgery or chemotherapy. Besides, evidence shows that consuming the standard American diet (SAD) actually feeds the cancer cells and tumors as we try to shrink them. The typical American diet includes various meats, dairy products, refined carbohydrates, processed sugar, and saturated fats.

I know in my heart that my plant-rich diet, along with carefully researched supplements, has been an important addition to my conventional treatments. This type of approach also has allowed me to survive and live more than 12 years after my diagnosis of this deadly sarcoma.

Conventional medicine has been slow to embrace current and past research concerning the link between the Western diet and cancer. Additionally, some medical authorities have voiced concerns about the type of nutritional information and guidance given to cancer patients by medical centers.

Patients and clinicians alike need to understand that certain types of food stuffs, along with the standard American diet, can lead to and encourage metastasis and shorter survival times. They need to understand that each patient's nutritional needs are very unique and need to be personalized. The links between poor nutrition (SAD) and survival outcomes are becoming more overt and need to be addressed early on during one's diagnosis. Moreover, sound anticancer nutrition may help address critical factors such as acidic environments, angiogenesis, inflammation, and compromised immune systems.

The mission of this chapter is twofold. The first is to help you understand the dire consequences of the standard American diet and lifestyle as it relates to cancer. Second, it is to guide you toward safer, healthier choices that may help save your life. It is my hope that through reading my story, you'll be better able to understand how to use nutrition to attack targets such as angiogenesis, inflammation, and your compromised immune system. Furthermore, eating a healthy, modified plant-based diet may even affect the environment inside and outside the tumor.

Confusion on the Front Lines

Month after month over the past decade, I have received phone calls from cancer patients across the United States seeking my advice about nutrition. I often hear a familiar theme during the course of the conversation: "My doctor told me to eat anything I want" or "They want me to do anything I can to sustain or gain weight."

Let's take a look at the current research and data coming out of the major cancer centers across the United States. *Cancer patients looking for dietary information online often find contradictory, inconsistent advice and an overall lack of information, even from the websites of top cancer centers,* according to a study by researchers at Thomas Jefferson University in Philadelphia. Only four of the top 21 websites of the National Comprehensive Cancer Network member institutions gave nutritional guidelines for patients during treatment.[8]

This study is not surprising, for two reasons. Number one, a significant percentage of cancer patients are given very little nutritional advice at all from their clinician or oncologist. Number two, these clinicians have very little education or training in anticancer nutrition and supplements. The bottom line is that each pa-

8. Nick Mulcahy, "Online Nutritional Advice for Cancer Patients is Scattershot," Medscape, March 23, 2013, http://www.medscape.com/viewarticle/781706.

tient needs a unique, customized, nutritional approach to their specific medical needs and tumor type. Additionally, they need an approach that will address inflammation, angiogenesis, and their immune status.

Renowned nutrition researchers T. Colin Campbell, PhD, and Thomas M. Campbell II, MD, write in their book *The China Study* that despite the public's hunger for information about nutrition, the contradictory and confusing data that the media sends out daily leaves them with endless questions.

> Given the barrage of information, are you confident that you know what you should be doing to improve your health? Should you buy food that is labeled organic to avoid pesticide exposure? Do carbohydrates really make you fat? What vitamins, if any, should you be taking? . . . My guess is that you're not really sure of the answers to these questions. If this is the case, then you aren't alone . . .
>
> This isn't because research hasn't been done. It has. We have an enormous amount about the links between nutrition and health. But the real science has been buried beneath a clutter of irrelevant or even harmful information—junk science, fad diets, and food industry propaganda.

Reading Dr. Campbell's book helped me enormously to understand the link between meat, dairy products, and cancer. His data and evidence linking the overabundance of animal protein with cancer was quite strong, in my opinion.

We need to have an honest discussion about how the standard American diet is contributing to epidemics like metabolic syndrome (diabetes, hypertension, and obesity), cancer, arthritis, and other chronic illnesses. We need to transform the way we practice healthcare by taking nutrition and lifestyle seriously.

Again, I want to note that a stressful lifestyle, combined with the typical American diet, often leads to life-threatening illnesses, such as diabetes, cardiovascular disease, and cancer. Unfortunately, most of us don't realize that we are killing ourselves. And more importantly, how do we stop this?

Problems with the American Diet

According to the World Health Organization, there is a tidal wave of cancer currently spreading around the globe, including in the United States. Moreover, there are strong links between the Western lifestyle, the standard American diet, and many malignancies. Furthermore, the epidemic of metabolic syndrome has been strongly implicated in many types of cancers and poor survival outcomes.

Studies show that people who eat large amounts of red meat have an increased risk of mortality. A study of more than 121,000 doctors and nurses, published in the *Archives of Internal Medicine* in 2012, found that those who ate a three-ounce serving of red meat each day were 13 percent more likely to die of cardiovascular disease or cancer. This number increased to 20 percent when participants ate processed meat more than once a day.

Tumor cell survival is dependent upon adaptation to acidic conditions in the tumor microenvironment, according to researchers at Moffitt Cancer Center and colleagues at the University of South Florida and Wayne State University. Their research, published in *Science Daily* in 2012, suggests that a successful treatment strategy might be based on leveraging this dependence. Cancer survivors can do their part by reducing the amount of acid forming foods in their diet, along with consuming certain vegetables that might increase their pH.

Sugar Is a Primary Fuel for Cancer

Let's talk about positron emission tomography, better known as PET scans. PET scans are actually computed tomography, or CAT scans, that are done approximately one hour after a patient is injected with radioactive glucose solution. Cancerous lesions of a certain size light up so that the radiologist can assess the patient's primary tumor, along with any metastasis or spread. These events happen because cancer cells have a rabid appetite for higher levels of insulin and glucose than normal cells.

Scientists at the University of California San Diego School of Medicine conducted a study to explore how consuming red meat can activate cancer growth. The 2010 study led by Dr. Ajit Varki suggests a sugar glycan molecule (Neu5Gc), which is introduced to the body through ingesting red meat, causes an inflammatory response. Because Neu5Gc appears to be foreign to the body, it creates antibodies against it. All this can cause inflammation, and chronic inflammation is a precursor of tumors.

It's well documented that obesity is a causative factor in diabetes, which occurs when the body fails to control sugar levels. High blood sugar not only contributes to these illnesses, it's also linked to increased cancer risk, according to a study published in 2013, led by Dr. Custodia Garcia-Jimenez at the University of Rey Juan Carlos in Madrid, Spain. He and his team found that high sugar levels trigger increased activity of a gene widely implicated in cancer progression.

Early on after my diagnosis, I started researching the Glycemic Index (GI) and Glycemic Load (GL). I wanted a diet that included foods that had low to moderate scores on these scales. Since insulin and glucose are two of cancer's main substrates (fuel), it only made sense to consume low glycemic foods.

The GI is used to tell you how quickly the carbohydrates in a particular food will raise your blood sugar. A number value is assigned to give a food a GI, and the higher the value, the more quickly the carbs from a certain food will raise your blood sugar. The GI does not include how many carbs are in a serving of a specific food, which is why knowing the GL of a food can offer more advantages. The GL includes both the GI and how many carbs are in a single serving of that food.

Studies tell us that eating foods with a high GI and a high GL could increase the risk of a variety of cancers, including breast, colorectal, lung, ovarian, and pancreatic.

According to a study published July 25, 2012 in *Annals of Oncology*, people may increase their risk for a number of cancers by eating high GI food or eating food with high GL. Research led by J. Hu of Centre for Chronic Disease Prevention and Control in 2012 found that GI was associated with the risk of prostate cancer. The study also found that eating high amounts of sugar, or a diet with high GL, was associated with a 28, 44, and 41 percent greater likelihood of developing colorectal cancer, rectal cancer, and pancreatic cancer respectively.

Various studies on high GL and GI diets and their association with breast cancer risk show contradictory results. Researchers say it's a result of difficulties inherent in measuring and analyzing this risk factor. Overall, the results from a number of 2012 studies show that normal weight women may be more susceptible to high glycemic diets. Some studies have found that women who consume a lot of sweets and sweet desserts have a higher risk for breast cancer. This includes a study in China of 74,942 women ages 40-70, who researchers followed for 7.35 years. Women in the highest quintile of GL had 1.45 times the risk of breast cancer as those in the lowest quintile.[9]

Again, women fighting breast cancer have to understand the importance of a low glycemic diet. Anticancer nutrition is the one thing that can not only help you feel a sense of control and empowerment, but can actually change the outcome of your disease.

A Cancer-Friendly versus Cancer-Unfriendly Environment
Many of us who are living a stressful lifestyle don't realize we are building a cancer-friendly environment. This means that our bodies are making certain hormones, chemicals, and cells that may accumulate into a malignancy. Furthermore, these small tumors want and need higher levels of insulin, glucose, and other substrates to grow.

---

9. "High Glycemic Load Diet Increses Risk of Breast Cncer," FoodforBreastCancer.com, http://foodfor-breastcancer.com/articles/high-glycemic-load-diet-increases-risk-of-breast-cancer.

In Dr. David Servan-Schrieber's book, *Anticancer*, he describes the difficulty in reversing a cancer-friendly environment. He writes, "As we have seen, while cancer can be triggered by any number of factors, it can only develop and spread if the terrain is favorable. There is no way to prevent cancer or slow down its growth (once it has already taken root) without changing this terrain in-depth."

Each of us has three basic terrains that we have to look at when we are diagnosed with cancer: 1.) biological/physical; 2.) emotional; and 3.) spiritual. These terrains are all interconnected and can profoundly affect each other. Consuming the SAD diet, along with feeling chronically stressed, often leads to inflammation and blockages, along with a more acidic environment. Additionally, if a person's mind and soul are not nourished, their body becomes a potential host for a variety of malignancies. Thus, we have a cancer-friendly terrain.

The answer is to slowly turn the situation around and learn how to heal yourself physically, emotionally, and spiritually. This often leads to creating a new anticancer terrain in your emotional and spiritual self, as well as in your body.

There are many factors that contribute to shaping a cancer-friendly terrain, including stress, lack of sleep, inflammation, and advanced age. As we age, the chances of triggering genetic aberrations inside us increase. Critical drivers of a cancer-friendly terrain include a sedentary lifestyle and the SAD diet. In *Cancer's Nature-Fighting Foods*, author Verne Varona writes, "Our modern diet of refined foods laden with chemicals and deficient in nutrients is currently thought to be the greatest single contributor to cancer development." He continues by discussing how dietary habits in the West have shifted from whole, natural foods to processed, convenience foods.

Varona outlines the following changes that have occurred over the past century: increased refined sugar, decreased whole grains; increased animal proteins, decreased vegetable proteins; increased saturated fats, decreased unsaturated fats; increased fiber-absent foods, decreased whole-fibrous foods; increased artificial additives, decreased naturally nutritious foods; increased synthetic chemicals, decreased natural quality; and increased fast-paced lifestyle, decreased meal-time rituals.

I think Varona is on to something. A plethora of research has come out in the past decade implicating these trends as some of the major causes of serious illnesses, including diabetes, heart disease, and cancer.

Food Became My Medicine

Lying in my hospital bed, I knew out of the gate that I would have to target this malignancy from many different avenues. I learned I would have to cut out most meats, dairy products, and sugar. I asked my friends and colleagues to bring me evidence-based anticancer books and research on nutrition. And interestingly, someone in my family helped me in a very unusual way: through a dream.

Looking back into my family history, I can honestly tell you that I had integrative medicine implanted in my genes. My maternal grandfather was named Floyd Wonser. He married my grandmother Margaret and they shared a wonderful, magical farm in Battle Creek, Michigan. Floyd did not have a need for much formal education, but he read a lot and became a wise, old soul.

When my grandmother died in the early 1990s, he took a great interest in holistic medicine out of a desire to increase his longevity. He started asking me to bring him books on natural and holistic medicine so he could create and implement his own regimens. Over time, he developed his own nutrition and exercise program, implementing a plant-based, nondairy diet that included natural supplements and bike riding. He lived many days past his original prognosis of congestive heart failure, dying in 2001 at age 99.

About four weeks after my original diagnosis in December of 2002 (I was very ill), my grandfather came to me in a dream. I could see his face, his brown eyes, and his grey-brown hair. He told me, "Mark, don't buy into the death sentences. You can live if you do the right things." He then went on to describe a nutrition program and supplements that he thought would help—a plant-rich diet, with occasional fish and healthy nuts. He went on to suggest apples, berries, and pomegranate. Additionally, he advised me to supplement with wheatgrass, vitamin C, and crushed flax meal.

I could feel the love, wisdom, and compassion coming from him that night, just as I could in the previous decades when he was alive. I have followed his advice from that night on, and it has made all the difference in my survival.

As I stated before, many of the experts I had seen around the country were not happy with my modified, plant-rich diet, or my consumption of natural supplements while I was off chemotherapy. Additionally, many of them warned me that this protocol would increase my demise and shorten my survival time. Their warnings were mind-boggling to me. As a matter of fact, very few of them offered any sound, evidence-based nutrition advice. Not only did they not address the critical gaps in conventional medicine, such as stopping inflammation or building my immune system, they were naïve of the fact that many studies show that most Americans consume a very deadly diet that is devoid of healthy fruits, vegetables, and phytonutrients.

I understood these issues from the outset and developed a plan of nutritional attack on my tumors from multiple fronts. Figure 1 shows the basis of the diet I adopted when I was diagnosed with cancer. I felt the need to make a dramatic change to ensure my survival. I created a generally plant-rich diet that occasionally incorporated fish or organic poultry. Every other day, I was strictly vegetarian.

To address inflammation, I consumed the following foods: citrus fruits, such as lemons and limes; leafy greens, such as kale, spinach, and watercress; and tomatoes. The fish included wild-caught salmon and cod. I put anticancer herbs on most meals, including basil, oregano, and thyme, and I added spices, such as cinnamon, ginger, and turmeric. I also consumed a large amount of beans, which are full of fiber and omega-3 fatty acids. Large amounts of fiber help to regulate blood sugar.

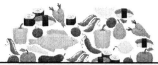

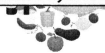

Figure 1—Mark Roby's Anticancer Diet

- High consumption of fiber based foods, such as vegetables and low-glycemic fruit.

- High consumption of legumes (such as beans, lentils, peas, and alfalfa)

- High consumption of nuts and seeds

- High consumption of anticancer herbs and spices (such as garlic, onion, turmeric, ginger, mustard)

- Modest consumption of complex carbohydrates (avoid processed foods and simple/refined carbohydrates)

- Modest consumption of healthy proteins (such as egg whites and the plant-based proteins pea, wheat germ, quinoa, and spirulina)

- Modest consumption of wild-caught fish (such as salmon, halibut, and red snapper)

- Low to modest consumption of organic turkey and chicken

- Low consumption of multiple whole grains (such as oatmeal, brown rice, whole wheat, barley)

- Replace dairy products with almond milk, rice milk, organic soy milk, and green, leafy vegetables

- Replace tap water with filtered or alkaline water

Additionally, I frequently consumed a concoction of wheat germ and flax meal to address inflammation and help stabilize my blood sugar.

To combat angiogenesis (blood supply to the tumor), I made a number of smoothies. One of my recipes included kale, apples, tomatoes, and pomegranate. Another was made up of pumpkin, blueberries, and strawberries. I often added filtered water or almond milk. I also consumed organic whey shakes with super greens (barley greens, wheatgrass, and other dark-green leafy vegetables) to build my glutathione levels and reduce inflammation. Glutathione is a natural antioxidant made by our livers that is a potent cancer fighter.

Day after day, night after night, week after week, I would juice and make smoothies with my blender. To increase my fiber intake, I added flax meal. Snacks included nuts, such as almonds, walnuts, or pistachios, because those have been shown to lower inflammation and reduce the lipid profile. I also grazed on low glycemic (sugars) fruits, such as apples, blueberries, and raspberries. I tried to avoid high sugar foods, such as starches, bananas, and potatoes. From my research, I knew that cancer's main fuel was glucose, which produces insulin and substrates that cause inflammation, from foods like red meat, dairy, etc. I stayed away from meat in general, along with yogurt, dairy products, and sweets.

Adding the Right Supplements

Following the first 12 to 15 months of my diagnosis, I thought it was extremely important to address my immune status. Again, when I asked my many oncologists how to strengthen the terrain of my immune system, they told me to take a multivitamin. This concerned me because I was often on chemo, had cachexia, and was exhausted most of the time. I knew that a multivitamin wasn't going to do it, and their lack of experience and knowledge regarding nutrition bothered me immensely. I wanted to tackle my symptoms, along with angiogenesis and inflammation, which cancer patients can deal with naturally.

I then went to my integrative medical doctor and requested an immune assay (blood work to assess the relative health of one's immune system) be ordered. My white blood cell count was chronically low, as were a few other components of my immune system. I also had my vitamin D-3 level checked and it was around 19, which was very low. Vitamin D-3 is a necessary component of a healthy immune system and can be taken as a supplement.

To build my immune system, I wanted to make sure that I consumed a colorful variety of vegetables and fruit. I knew that if I ate veggies, like dark leafy greens, red and green peppers, and the occasional sweet potatoes, I would be building my immune system and supplying myself with healthy nutrients and vitamins. I wanted to fill myself with as many phytonutrients as I could. I wanted to detoxify my body, address angiogenesis, and reduce inflammation.

After numerous discussions on the phone and in person with my integrative medical doctor, we came up with the following regimen while I was off chemotherapy:

- Resveratrol (antioxidant and anti-inflammatory with antiproliferative effects in clinical trials)

- Green tea extract (antioxidant and e-acid, which inhibits inflammation and angiogenesis)

- Alpha lipoic acid (a vitaminlike substance that increases glutathione levels)

- Fish oil (anti-inflammatory)

- Wheatgrass (anti-inflammatory)

- Vitamin D-3 (anti-inflammatory and antioxidant)

• Betasterols (anti-inflammatory)

• Intravenous vitamin C and glutathione infusions

This protocol was designed to help guide my inner terrain towards a cancer-unfriendly environment. Additionally, I wanted to make the tumor's microenvironment less hospitable to cancer.

Cancer-Fighting Foods

What are the ways in which you can make your inner terrain more cancer unfriendly? Let's look at some of the studies. Research conducted by the Angiogenesis Foundation proposes that you can stop cancer before it starts to grow, an approach they call "anti-angiogenesis." The thinking is that by changing the way you eat, you can change your "internal environment," and by doing so, you deprive cancer cells of their ability to grow. Certain foods, eaten in correct portions and frequency, can discourage cancer growth, including bok choy, cooked tomatoes, flounder, strawberries, and artichokes.[10]

A simple change in diet may significantly improve the survival of men with prostate cancer, according to a study led by the University of California, San Francisco that was published in *JAMA Internal Medicine* in 2013. It was found that by eating healthy vegetable fats, instead of animal fats and carbohydrates, men with prostate cancer had a much lower risk of developing lethal prostate cancer and dying from other causes. These healthy vegetable fats include olive and canola oil, nuts, seeds, and avocados.

Regularly consuming foods with a high concentration of flavonoids is associated with lower levels of insulin resistance and inflammation, based on a study by researchers at King's College London and the University of East Anglia in the *Journal of Nutrition*. These foods include berries, chocolate, herbs, red grapes, certain vegetables, and wine.

---

10. http://www.doctoroz.com/article/5-foods-starve-cancer.

Berries, in particular, contain two compounds—anthrocyanins and polyphenol ellagic acid—that may make them effective cancer fighters. In animal models of esophageal cancer, researchers have found at least seven berry types that help prevent cancer. They may each work a little differently, but they all seem to have a positive effect, according to Gary Stoner, PhD, professor of medicine at the Medical College of Wisconsin, who has studied the potential link of berries to cancer prevention for 20 years.[11]

Up to 40 percent of women ages 40-50 may have tiny cancers in their breasts, but the body's natural anticancer systems usually stop them from growing larger and becoming harmful.[12] Certain foods are thought to be anti-angiogenic, meaning they support the body's control of these cancerous cells. They include green tea, berries of different varieties, citrus fruits, apples, pineapple, cherries, red grapes, red wine, bok choy, kale, soybeans, ginseng, maitake mushrooms, licorice, turmeric, nutmeg, artichokes, lavender, pumpkin, sea cucumber, tuna, parsley, garlic, tomato, olive oil, grape seed oil, dark chocolate, and pomegranate.

I've consumed most of these foods out of the gate, and that has made all the difference. It's exciting and empowering to know that you can make a difference just by the actions you can take on your own. Your diet is one of the things that you can control.

The Power of a Plant-Rich Diet

Cancer patients have to start realizing that what they consume is just as important as any surgery or chemotherapy that they might receive. When they frequently ingest a diet that has a high GL, they are asking for trouble. It would behoove all of us with cancer to study and research ways to stabilize our blood sugar. Furthermore, there is talk of clinical trials in which cancer patients would go on a restricted calorie diet to see if that could increase survival times. Protocols such as a modified Mediterranean

11. American Institute for Cancer Research, "Berries: Sweetening Cancer Prevention," *ScienceNow* 41, Summer 2012, http://www.aicr.org/assets/docs/pdf/sciencenow/sciencenow-41.pdf.

12. "The Best Way to Prevent Cancer: A Good Diet," *O: The Oprah Magazine*, May 2010, http://www.oprah.com/health/Prevent-Cancer-with-the-Right-Diet-of-Antiangiogenic-Foods/print/1.

diet, high fiber foods, and vegetable proteins can assist us in these goals.

Speaking of anticancer diets, in her book *Zest for Life: The Mediterranean Anti-Cancer Diet*, nutrition expert Conner Middelmann-Whitney states:

> Over the millennia, the wide diversity of foods and flavors around the Mediterranean gave rise to markedly distinct and diverse culinary traditions. But what is striking is that almost every food thought to have anticancer properties—such as garlic, onions, cabbage, berries, green tea, mushrooms, olive oil, oily fish, nuts, seeds, lentils, aromatic herbs, spices, and a wide and colorful range of fruit and vegetables—is an integral part of the Mediterranean diet, no matter which region. From a purely biological perspective, in terms of the range and depth of nutrients it supplies, the pre-industrial Mediterranean diet is probably the closest thing to the optimal anti-cancer diet.

You don't have to go to Greece or Italy to adopt a Mediterranean diet. Instead of becoming strict vegetarians, I bet many cancer survivors could more easily adapt to the protocols I outlined in the diet I followed in Figure 1. Personally, I credit much of my survival to my plant-rich diet. I also think it's best for cancer patients to consume a vegetarian diet two to three days a week. Recent studies are showing stronger links between vegetables, fruit, nuts, and legumes and cancer-fighting properties.

While I do eat meat, it's in very small quantities and only occasionally. I cut out most meats and meat by-products. I eat wild, fatty fish, such as salmon, and small amounts of organic turkey and chicken. I also find high-quality protein in certain vegetables. For dairy, I substitute almond milk and organic soy products.

Figure 2 on the next page outlines the seven colors of health. It should help you, the patient, gain a better understanding of some of the properties of the Mediterranean diet. Visuals like this one really helped me early on to choose a nu-

Figure 2 — The Seven Colors of Health

Color & Active Phytonutrient	Food Sources	Physiological Functions
Red (lycopene)	Tomatoes, pink grapefruit, watermelon, processed tomatoes (tomato paste, ketchup, soup, juice)	Antioxidant, induces enzymes that protect cells against carcinogens; may protect against prostate and lung cancers
Red/Purple (antocyanidins, proanthocyanidins, ellagic acid)	Red apples, red peppers, blackberries, blueberries, red cabbage, cherries, cranberries or cranberry juice/sauce, eggplant, red grapes or juice, red pears, plums, pomegranates, prunes, strawberries, red wine	Antioxidant, anti-angiogenic, may help prevent the binding of carcinogens to DNA; may protect against gastro-intestinal cancers
Orange (alpha and beta carotenes)	Carrots, mangos, apricots, cantaloupes, pumpkin, acorn squash, winter squash, sweet potatoes	Antioxidant, may improve communication between cells; may help prevent lung cancer
Orange/Yellow (beta-crypothanxin, a minor carotenoid)	Orange juice, oranges, tangeries, peaches, papayas, nectarines	Antioxidant, may inhibit cholesterol synthesis needed to activate cancer cell growth
Yellow/Green (carotenoids lutein, zeaxanthin)	Avocados, peppers (green or yellow), collard greens, sweet corn, cucumber, green beans, honeydew melon, kiwifruit, mustard greens, peas, green romaine lettuce, spinach, turnip greens, zucchini (with skin)	Help correct DNA imbalances; help stimulate enzymes that break down carcinogens
Green (sulforaphane, isothiocyanate, indoles)	Broccoli, Brussels sprouts, bok choy, cabbage, cauliflower, kale, Swiss chard, watercress	Stimulate the release of enzymes that break down cancer-causing chemicals in the liver; may inhibit early tumor growth

Source: Conner Middelmann-Whitney, *Zest for Life: The Mediterranean Anti-Cancer Diet*

tritional attack on my tumor. Slowly, step by step, I learned to build a customized anticancer diet that is keeping me alive to this day. Furthermore, many patients I counsel who follow this approach are doing remarkably well. Each of them is following a unique, personalized plan that is right for them.

Unbeknownst to many Americans, plants such as fruits and vegetables can often counteract the deadly side effects of the SAD diet. Furthermore, a modified plant-based diet may help individuals prevent obesity, cardiovascular disease, and cancer. These foods don't just provide vitamins, minerals, and fiber, they add phytochemicals, which may boost the immune system, fight infection, and protect against cancer, as Middelmann-Whitney suggests. Consuming a wide variety of colorful fruits and vegetables is essential for building a healthy inner terrain. Additionally, these phytochemicals may help prevent inflammation and angiogenesis, which are two hallmarks of cancer.

The Benefits of Integrative Medicine

There is a growing demand for integrative medicine and evidence-based nutrition among cancer patients in the United States. Integrative medicine is the use of non-invasive, safe techniques and modalities, such as nutrition, meditation, yoga, and acupuncture as an adjunct to conventional medicine. It may also include other modalities, such as guided imagery, stress reduction, and natural supplements.

Cancer patients, like myself, constantly have to combat physical, emotional, psychological, and financial stress on a daily basis much more so than the average person. And scientific evidence shows that stress may escalate the growth of cancer tumors by increasing cortisone levels and recruiting inflammatory cells such as cytokines into their microenvironment. Below are some integrative methods I used to reduce stress after my diagnosis and still use today:

- Meditation

- Acupuncture

- Massage

- Yoga

- Guided imagery

Current research shows that modalities such as mindfulness, meditation, acupuncture, massage, and energy work may very well lower stress levels, minimize side effects, and increase feelings of well-being. Many of these protocols are not only safer than drugs and chemo, but there is little to no evidence that they are harmful in any way.

Unfortunately, many of these modalities that could help patients are not covered by insurance. Furthermore, a significant percentage of clinicians are not referring patients to integrative clinics housed in their own medical centers. What's concerning is that studies show a significant percentage of cancer patients do not discuss these options with their clinicians, either. And while many cancer patients are not talking to their doctors about integrative medicine, it doesn't mean they are not using it. Many patients are using these modalities, but they're hesitant to bring them up during their office visits.

Glenn Sabin, cancer survivor, discusses the growth in consumer use of integrative medicine in his blog:

> No doubt, health consumers have become savvier. The Internet has accelerated this pace . . . A growing army of consumers already understand their choices. They are voting with their choice of medical practitioners and the hospitals and centers where they have privileges . . . Organizations that ignore the growing consumer demand for integrative healthcare—and those shuttering existing programs as an austerity measure—do so at their own long-term economic peril.

I have to say, that based on my personal experience, if it weren't for integrative medicine and anticancer nutrition, I wouldn't be alive today.

Key Points

In order to survive, I knew I had to make significant changes to my diet and lifestyle out of the gate. I give as much credit to these changes for my survival as I do to the miracles of modern medicine. Anticancer nutrition, along with lifestyle changes, are critical lifelines for all cancer survivors.

Some of the key concepts that we covered in this chapter are:

- Your diet and lifestyle (related to your diagnosis and prognosis) are much more important than you are being told.

- The current recommendations and protocols coming out of medical centers are sometimes confusing and contradictory.

- Various meats, dairy products, sugars, refined carbohydrates, and saturated fat may contribute to a poor prognosis and shorter survival times.

- Slowly, purposefully turning your terrain from cancer-friendly to cancer-unfriendly is crucial for your survival.

Lifelines/Action Steps

Anticancer nutrition is an important adjunct that should always be used alongside conventional therapy. The following are actions you can take to become cancer whole:

- Become more conscious of your diet and lifestyle

- Consider following a modified, personalized Mediterranean diet, which can help you to achieve your goals

- Study and research the foods that combat inflammation and angiogenesis, as they may help strengthen your terrain against cancer and other diseases

- Work with your naturopath, integrative clinician, or nutritionist to consume nutrients that will boost your immune system and lower your glycemic load

In addition, here are some websites you can visit:

- ***American Institute of Cancer Research*** (www.aicr.org) is an anticancer resource center that offers cancer prevention and research information. It includes anticancer recipes and a nutrition hotline.

- ***Angiogenesis Foundation*** (www.angio.org) is an excellent evidence-based site where you can find articles and videos concerning the role of nutrition and diet as they relate to angiogenesis.

- ***Eat to Beat Cancer*** (www.eattobeatcancer.org) is a website designed to improve health through cancer-fighting foods. It offers cutting-edge, evidence-based nutrition information.

- ***CANCERactive*** (http://www.canceractive.com) is where you'll find a plethora of information about integrative oncology, nutrition, and newer conventional techniques (such as vaccines and more).

- ***Harvard Health Publications*** (http://www.health.harvard.edu/healthy-eating/glycemic_index_and_glycemic_load_for_100_foods) from the Harvard Medical School has information on the Glycemic Index and Glycemic Load, including easy to read charts.

I also suggest you take a look at the following books:

- *Zest for Life: The Mediterranean Anti-Cancer Diet* by Conner Middelmann-Whitney (www.zestforlife.com)

- *Foods to Fight Cancer: Essential Foods to Help Prevent Cancer* by Richard Beliveau, PhD

- *Nature's Cancer-Fighting Foods* by Verne Varona, an excellent groundbreaking read written by a very wise author

- *The After Cancer Diet*, an e-book by Suzanne Boothby

Here are several cancer coaches or guides with whom you can consult:

- Conner Middelmann-Whitney, a nutritionist, health writer, and cooking instructor, is a cancer survivor who can work with you personally to customize your diet (www.modernmediterranean.com).

- Susan Gonzalez, RN, BSN, a cancer survivor, author, and nutrition expert, has a book on nutrition and health tips to help people survive cancer and is a great resource (http://100perksofhavingcancer.com/).

- Dr. Shani Fox, ND, whose signature system "Beyond a 'New Normal': Your Guide to Getting Back in Charge and Creating Extraordinary Wellness and Joy after Cancer" nurtures deep wellness and body-mind harmony that increases resilience to disease, is an expert in anticancer nutrition (http://www.drshanifox.com/).

Summary

The standard american diet (SAD) is not only dangerous, studies show it's connected to many common cancers. It's essential you understand these links between the Western diet and cancer drivers, such as inflammation and angiogenesis, and realize that obesity and poor dietary habits may lead to a poor prognosis. According to research, understanding the benefits of a modified Mediterranean diet, Glycemic Index, and Glycemic Load is crucial. Working with these concepts can make your physical terrain (your body) cancer-unfriendly.

> *"You can rise above this.*
> *There is a way through it.*
> *You can survive."*
> — Mark Roby

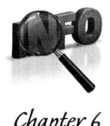

Chapter 6

Lifelines to Research

"Cancer is a biological problem, not a statistical problem."
— Anonymous

"Nothing in life is to be feared, only understood."
— Marie Curie

Sandy Barker's back was up against the wall. It was May 2006, on her son's birthday, that Christian walked past her looking pale and fatigued, with huge bruises all over him. She took him to his doctor, who performed some tests. The next day she received an urgent call to get her son to the emergency room immediately for more testing. The answers came the following day.

The doctor told us that Christian had pre-B cell acute lymphoblastic leukemia (ALL) type cancer. Our lives were changed forever. While I suspected this diagnosis, I don't think any parent is ever ready to hear "Your child has cancer." Time stands still. The words echo in your ears. You have to remind yourself to breathe. You pray it is all a bad dream. Then when you realize it isn't, the tears start flowing uncontrollably and you cry out to God!!

The prognosis was grim, so Sandy and her husband decided to quickly enroll Christian in a clinical trial.

> Two weeks after Christian started receiving his chemo, we were given more horrible news by his doctor. With a heavy heart, Christian's doctor told us that after further testing, Christian's cancer has a cytogenetic involvement called Hypodiploid Acute Lymphoblastic Leukemia. He said it is a very rare, aggressive, and resistant cancer, and that he had only seen it four times in the 27 years he had been practicing. Furthermore, he explained that Christian had to be taken off the clinical trial, and he needed a bone marrow transplant.

Sandy contacted 10 major medical centers and chose Seattle Cancer Care Alliance to perform the grueling bone marrow transplant (BMT) on Christian. After 100 days, he seemed home free. But two months later, the cancer returned, and the only option left was another bone marrow transplant. Christian bravely went through his second transplant, yet it did not stave it off, either. He then developed graft versus host disease (GVHD). Things looked grim, and his only hope for survival was an experimental drug called Prochymal®. Sandy and her doctors petitioned the FDA and hospital to escalate the process and obtain approval. Unfortunately, there were delays and Christian continued to decline each day.

> On Christmas day 2007 Christian coded, and we were told his liver was failing from the effects of the GVHD. We signed DNR (do not resuscitate) papers on Christmas morning instead of opening gifts as a family. My little warrior hung on for five more days, and went to heaven just before midnight on December 29, 2007, with our family by his side whispering in his ears: "We love you! We are so proud of you!!"

I will never forget watching Christian take his last breath at the age of 14 and a half. The thought of that is still difficult for us. Christian died cancer-free, from complications of GVHD. No child or family should have to endure what Christian and our family did. There must be more effective and less toxic options! This is the verse we wrote on Christian's website the night he died. I feel it applies to all of the heroic angels who fought like Christian did and are angels now. *"I have fought the good fight, I have finished the race, I have kept the faith. There is in store for me the crown of righteousness, which the Lord, the righteous Judge, will award to me on that day." — 2 Timothy 4: 7-8*

Sandy spends many days and weeks going to Washington, D.C. advocating for the many children like her son. She speaks to congressmen, senators, and the Food and Drug Administration (FDA), pushing for safer, more therapeutic options for these children. Sandy and her husband founded a nonprofit called The Gold Rush Cure Foundation, which helps mentor parents and assists children in fighting cancer in a variety of ways. You can find Christian's full story and information on the foundation on Sandy's website (www.goldrush.org).

Are You Taking the Right First Steps?
This gripping story exemplifies the plight of many adults and children facing unusual or aggressive malignancies. They may be offered very limited options, which they use up in a short amount of time.

As a cancer patient, you may be the perfect role model: compliant, dedicated, and doing everything you are told. Then, disaster strikes. Patients can do all they are told, but to no avail. For many cancer patients, parents of children with cancer, and researchers, the limited options are frustrating.

In "World War Cancer," an article by Alexander Nazaryan, published in *The New Yorker* magazine in June 2013, Nazaryan discusses author/survivor Clifton

Leaf. He describes Leaf's book, *The Truth in Small Doses: Why We Are Losing the War on Cancer and How to Win It,* as follows:

> Leaf argues we should be closer to an all-out cure, considering our invest-ment in the effort . . . In Leaf's telling, oncology is a hideout field averse to risk, a culture that "has grown progressively less hospitable to new voices and ideas over the past four decades."

My question to you is, Do you really know what you are up against? Furthermore, do you and your oncologist know the secrets of your specific tumor and its meta-bolic response to potential treatments? *Many times, the answer to both of these questions is "no."* That's why you must take charge and find the individuals and laboratories that will give you the crucial answers that may save your life and save you from toxic, deadly side effects.

The current standard of care often does not include molecular profiling, chemosensitivity assays, personalized vaccines, or anticancer nutrition. It is my hope that with these tools, cancer patients will find the genetic secrets to their tumor, along with the tumor's response to potentially lifesaving therapies. In addition, they can use integrative medicine modalities to make their own body more cancer-unfriendly.

Asking for More Personalized Treatment

In March 2004 I returned home from my four-week stay at the Immune Institute in southern California. During my time there I received many natural IVs, and learned yoga and meditation along with other nutritional modalities that strength-ened my immune system and made my body more cancer-unfriendly.

At home, my scans revealed that these adjuncts had slowed my tumor growth down to a crawl. Yet a subsequent scan three months later revealed new tumors in my liver. So I decided to make the rounds at three large cancer centers I had visited previously.

For the second time in a 15-month span, my efforts were fruitless. In fact, one of the associate directors of a prestigious cancer center said, "Mark, why do you keep coming back? We told you the last time that there's nothing we can do for you." I begged him to research my tumor and put me in clinical trials. I told him I had run out of options. "Mark," he retorted, "we told you last time that researching your tumor and doing a molecular profile was of no clinical relevance."

I found out later that this was the furthest thing from the truth. Additionally, he told me that my nutritional program and integrative strategies were dangerous and could speed my demise. I left his office discouraged, hopeless, and downtrodden.

A short time later, I met a woman at Gilda's Club (national cancer support network) with advanced breast cancer, who was seeing an integrative medical doctor. He was assisting her in obtaining a less toxic European chemo treatment called Ukrain. It was a non-FDA approved medicine that was not covered by insurance and was very expensive. It worked in a similar manner to thalidomide (a specialized chemotherapy) and had been used in Europe for various sarcomas.

Her story sparked my interest, and about two months later my friends and colleagues had raised more than $9,000 for me, enough to cover the treatment for approximately three to four months. My colleagues actually risked their own licenses and livelihoods to administer this treatment to me behind closed doors in their offices, kitchens, and living rooms. The therapy did, indeed, stabilize my tumors, and after nine months, there was a slight regression in some of them. This therapy was very helpful in keeping me alive for almost a year, while the medical establishment had given up on me.

Over the next few years, I spent most of my free time researching the nuances of the type of sarcoma I had. I found out that its growth is often slow, but can become rapid. Furthermore, it was a very vascular tumor that often metastasized from the liver to the lungs or bones. To keep myself alive, my treatments alternated between the Ukrain therapy and Avastin.

Between 2006 and 2007, my condition worsened and my liver tumors started growing more rapidly. My research helped guide me to a fellow sarcoma patient, Avi, a businessman who lives in New Jersey. He and his wife introduced me to his renowned oncologist at Columbia Presbyterian Medical Center in New York City, who had helped get his cancer into partial remission. This specialist enrolled me in a clinical trial studying the effects of a new drug called Sutent®. This agent is a multikinase inhibitor that was initially used for a specific type of kidney cancer.

Columbia Presbyterian Hospital was an essential lifeline for me in that they did everything they could to keep me alive until my liver transplant in 2009. They actually took my research seriously and allowed me to use a shared decision-making approach with them to drive my care. Furthermore, they did not discourage me from using my plant-rich diet or my carefully researched natural supplements. I could not have survived without their open-minded, personalized approach.

Eventually, this agent kept me alive and stabilized my tumors for two and a half years. I am so grateful for the generosity and skills of my physician there and his renowned medical center, along with the Attitudinal Healing Center, Michelle Phaump (founder and president of Lend a Helping Hand), and my colleagues for their fundraising efforts that allowed me to travel.

Turning the Tide

Are you exhausted, anxious, and confused concerning your diagnosis and treatment? Have you recently been given a poor prognosis or a questionable treatment plan? How do you know if your current or next treatment regimen is going to work and carry you safely through the storm?

I know what it's like to be frightened out of your mind. I also remember what it was like to feel trapped and running out of options. I can recall that time like it was yesterday . . . the anxiety, the panic, and the sleepless nights I went through, especially in the first three to four months after my diagnosis. During those periods, I would go somewhere alone and pray for guidance or signs.

Here are some actions you can take to keep you afloat:

- Become informed and engaged, which could lead you to better and safer choices regarding your survival.

- Educate yourself about the basics of cancer and your tumor type, which could help keep you alive and safe.

- Seek out resources, such as top-flight oncologists, researchers, and mentors (fellow cancer survivors) who could help you tilt the balance from death toward life.

- Learn about cutting-edge research, such as "The Hallmarks of Cancer" (important, scientific, peer reviewed), that can increase your understanding of molecular profiling and may help you obtain safer, more targeted therapies.

- Implement integrative medicine into your regimen. It may help you to attack your tumors from multiple fronts, including with regard to inflammation and angiogenesis, which are part of the tumor microenvironment.

These actions helped me to create my Triad of Survival/contingency plans four times over, gave me safer treatments, and kept me alive.

Be Prepared for Challenges
There are countless patients who walk into their specialist's office daily after researching their cancer diagnosis, looking for personalized treatments. They are also

looking for safer, more effective options for saving their lives. Yet at times, their requests can be met with resistance.

Consider the following story of one patient who asked about a chemosensitivity assay. It comes from the book *Customized Cancer Treatment* by Ralph Moss, PhD. Dr. Moss shares a letter written to him by one of his readers who accompanied her sister on an appointment to her oncologist. While there, her sister requested a special type of testing for her tumor, called a chemosensitivity and resistant assay. This test potentially could lead to safer, more effective therapies. The doctor's response was less than desirable.

> This morning, during our appointment with my sister's oncologist, we brought this possibility to the attention of her doctor. We were BLASTED all the way up and down, as if we were committing a crime of cosmic proportion. The doctor was so mad. You cannot imagine the scene. We were alone, trying to treat my sister with something better, and every time we try something new, we are blasted like this. And I know we are not alone. If you elaborate more, many people can take advantage of our sad experience, and maybe you can give us more elements to fight back.

Patients like this motivated Dr. Moss to write his book, *Customized Cancer Care*, for people who want to try something new but are shut down by medical providers. If I had not researched my own diagnosis, carefully vetted my doctors, and armed myself with cutting-edge data, ***I would not have had a chance at survival. Cancer patients are putting their lives at risk if they are simply quiet, complacent, and subservient*** without partnering with clinicians and others in their own care. To survive, it is your job to talk to your clinician about these new approaches called "lifelines." Your life could depend upon it.

TOM ALLEN

Tom Allen is a gifted and talented musician and engineer whom I met at church. After one Sunday service, he confided to me that he'd recently been diagnosed with esophageal cancer. He explained the stress he was under concerning many important medical decisions that he was facing. A short time later, Tom came to see me in my office. We discussed a personalized anticancer diet, multiple opinions, the risks and benefits of each surgical procedure, and more.

What impressed me was that despite his fear and stress, Tom was not the typical cancer patient. He was engaged, informed, and empowered. He made every decision carefully. Often Tom would step back, research his options, and analyze the implications.

Like so many people who find themselves in a crisis, Tom centered himself by writing about his cancer journey. Here is an excerpt from his own journal:

After I was diagnosed, I immediately began researching my condition. Being a research engineer by trade, I was good at this. I spent hours on the Internet reading about esophageal cancer. Not much was encouraging: the five year survival rates were pretty low.

I needed to get a port installed on my body for the chemo. The port would direct the chemo directly into a vein. Apparently, injecting it into one's arm is not the optimal approach. This required surgery, so I was apprehensive about it, but I researched the procedure online and this made me somewhat less fearful.

All my research really helped reduce my anxiety about the treatments. There are all sorts of horror stories about chemo and its side effects. The radiation machine looks menacing. Someone who didn't know about the chemistry of chemo or the technology involved in radiation could easily feel uncomfortable and anxious. But when I started these treatments, I knew a lot about them. I had little fear.

Then, I faced what was perhaps the most important decision of life. My options were a choice between two complicated surgeries or simply sticking with chemo and radiation. Each decision had different possible risks and benefits, and I had to weigh the safety and efficacy of each. In the end, it was research and talking to other patients that helped me the most.

To read Tom Allen's full story, visit www.LifelinestoCancerSurvival.com.

Tools for Researching Your Own Diagnosis

There are a number of important research tools that many patients don't know about, including *molecular profiling, cancer biomarkers,* and *chemosensitivity assays.* Additionally, *TumorGrafts* implanted in *animal surrogates,* along with *personalized vaccines,* could be potentially lifesaving.

Molecular profiling, as defined by the Mayo Clinic, is a method of testing that examines each person's cancer tumor and studies the genetic characteristics, as well as any unique biomarkers. The information gathered is used to identify and create targeted therapies that are designed to work better for a specific cancer tumor profile.

Speaking from my own experience, molecular profiling saved my life. Pathologists at a major medical center found a growth pathway called mTOR in my tumor that guided my liver transplant team to put me on a drug called Rapamune® (mTOR inhibitor) that is keeping my liver cancer-free.

Biomarkers can refer to many different compounds in the body that indicate something about your health. There are biomarkers for heart disease, multiple sclerosis, and many other diseases. When people talk about cancer biomarkers, they're usually referring to proteins, genes, and other molecules that affect how cancer cells grow, multiply, die, and respond to other compounds in the body.

While some cancer biomarkers can be used to predict how aggressively your cancer will grow, and are therefore useful for prognosis, the most promising use of biomarkers today is to identify which therapies a particular patient's cancer may or may not respond to. Cancer biomarkers★ can include:

- Proteins

- Gene mutations

- Gene rearrangements

- Extra copies of genes

- Missing genes

- Other molecules

★ *Biomarker information courtesy of http://www.mycancer.com*

A *chemosensitivity assay*, as defined by the National Cancer Institute, is a laboratory test that measures the number of tumor cells killed by a particular cancer drug. Tumor cells are removed from the body and then flown out that day to specialized labs. Once they arrive at the lab, the cells are exposed to older and then more advanced therapeutic agents to look for safer, more effective treatment options. So a chemosensitivity assay may help in choosing the best drug or drugs for the cancer being treated. Even though this test is seldom used, it has been a lifesaver for a number of my patients. It could be a critical lifeline for individuals with advanced, rare, or aggressive cancers.

Here are some other ways you can investigate your own cancer type and its microenvironment:

1 Talk to cancer center/medical center librarians (ask them to assist you in understanding the basics of your cancer type). This is my top choice.

2 **My Cancer Genome** (www.Mycancergenome.org) is a personalized cancer medicine resource for physicians, patients, and caregivers. The site gives up-to-date information on what makes cancers grow, along with therapeutic implications and available clinical trials. The site is managed by the Vanderbilt-Ingram Cancer Center.

3 For news bulletins and reports on significant issues regarding the current cancer landscape, see *Medical News Today* (http://www.medicalnewstoday.com/-categories/cancer-oncology). The site covers types, symptoms, causes, and treatments for cancer.

4 For breaking news on the diagnosis and treatment of cancer, with news feeds from all over the world, go to http://web2news.com/cancer.

5 Well known for providing solid, evidence-based medical information, *WebMD* will give you the basics on the symptoms, diagnosis, testing, and treatments for many types of cancer (http://www.webmd.com/breast-cancer/default.htm).

6 Go to the **National Cancer Institute** (NCI) website (http://www.cancer.gov/), where you'll find great information to assess the basics of your tumor and beyond.

7 Learn about the relationship between blood supply and tumor growth. The **Angiogensis Foundation** website (http://www.angio.org/) is one resource for more information.

8 Read magazines such as *Cure, Cancer World,* and *Cancer Today* that cover basic cancer information through cutting-edge research for the layperson.

9 Dr. Brian Rubin is a world-renowned pathologist and medical researcher who has made invaluable contributions to sarcoma diagnosis and treatment. The list of his more than 170 publications is impressive. During the last couple of years, Dr Rubin assumed a leadership role in the research of Epitheliod Hemangioendothelioma, one of the rarest sarcomas with no standard treatment. He discovered the disease's underlying genetic cause and identified potential targeted therapy for EHE and MEK inhibitors. The first rational-based clinical trial is on the way. If you would like to contribute to his research for rare sarcomas, go to http://giving.ccf.org/goto/EHEresearch.

Remember, you can take it one step at a time. Initially, learn the basics about cancer and the cancer cell. Start by reading books and articles about what fuels the cancer cell and your tumor. Going forward, there are many books and sites, including YouTube, that will teach you the basics of simple genetics. This will lead you towards learning about and understanding the molecular targets of your specific tumor type.

Driving Your Own Care

In this new frontier, *you* are the CEO of your life and care. *You* are the director. *You* are the final decision-maker. *You* must chart your own course. So how can you go about starting to understand your diagnosis and treatment plan? Start by reading websites, journals, and magazines about basic concepts concerning your diagnosis. If you are too sick or overwhelmed to do this, then you *must* find people who will do this for you. *You must learn how to become an engaged, informed patient.* Your life depends on it. Researching your own diagnosis is a critical lifeline in building your Triad of Survival. The wisdom and knowledge that you glean from this process may very well save your life. It is the sustenance and glue that will bring all of your lifelines together and keep you going.

The decision as to whether or not to research your own illness could make the difference between life and death. Over the past century, patients have given away their autonomy and left the research up to their clinician, trusting that they know everything there is to know. Today patients have access to advanced research and treatment options that the average person did not have access to in the past. There is no reason not to use all of the weapons at your disposal in the battle for your life.

Very, very few of the medical professionals I encountered had researched my specific tumor type in depth. *That's why it's your job to find out everything you can about your type of tumor or cancer.* You cannot leave it up to anyone else. I keep repeating this because it's becoming more evident through the latest scientific research that discovering your tumor's genetic fingerprint and the secrets of its microenvironment (inflammatory cells, blood vessel growth, other tissue, and nutrients surrounding your tumor) is imperative in saving your life. In an article entitled "Towards a Genetic Definition of Cancer-Associated Inflammation: Role of the IDO Pathway," published in the May 2010 edition of the *American Journal of Pathology*, authors George C. Prendergast, Richard Metz, and Alexander J. Muller state that " . . . beyond the cancer cell itself, it is clear that the tissue microenvironment exerts powerful effects in determining progression versus dormancy or destruction of an oncogenically initiated cell." I also know this to be true because I had to do a decade of research on my own tumor's microenvironment to keep myself alive.

Some of the oncologists I met were kind, sensitive people doing their best to help me. And your oncologist may be kind, sensitive, and doing his or her best, however, the standard of care often fails individuals facing difficult cancers. If you're facing a tough prognosis, it is *your* job to do your own research and do your best to get your clinician to buy into doing this research.

You don't have time to waste. Furthermore, you want to know if the clinicians or hospitals you contact are really engaged in new approaches to cancer survival.

You are looking for experts and institutions that are up to date with genetic profiling, potential chemosensitivity assays, and integrative medicine.

Once you have obtained a list of names through your research, the next step is to contact them by phone. Many clinical trial investigators and their staff will talk to you if you can get through their gatekeepers. A gatekeeper can be a specialist's secretary or a telephone triage nurse at a major cancer center. Oftentimes, they want to protect the clinicians and get you to come into their hospital or medical center. Your job is to get past them and start vetting the specialists or institutions to see if they meet your needs. Instead of calling their 800 number, call them directly at their office (find their specific number via the hospital information on the Internet or at your library). Ask your family doctor or any medical professional you know to make the call for you. Present yourself as a potential patient to discover if the doctor can help you or not.

If you are still unable to make direct contact with the specialist, speak to his or her nurses, nurse practitioners, or physician assistants. Flattery will get you everywhere. Tell the gatekeeper that you've read the doctor's research, books, and articles and really, really like what you see. Ask them if the doctor or mid-level practitioner could have a five-minute conversation with you. Tell them, "I'm up against the wall."

How do you truly know the risks and benefits of each procedure and treatment? The same way you get to Carnegie Hall (sort of): research, research, research. What are the benefits of researching your diagnosis? Each and every decision you make—based on that research—could have an impact on your survival time. The more informed and educated you are concerning your diagnosis and treatment plan, the better your chance of survival.

The benefits of doing all that research may include:

• Decreased anxiety and depression

• Increased feelings of well-being, safety, and hope

- Better, healthier nutrition, which could boost your immune system

- A potentially higher tier of medical care

- Learning the genetic target of your specific tumor, which could lead to a more customized, lifesaving treatment

- Safer, more effective treatment

- Learning how integrative medicine could attack certain targets or hallmarks of your tumor (i.e., inflammation and angiogenesis)

- Creating your own personal Triad of Survival that could save your life

Key Points

We are now roaming the new frontier of cancer care. As a cancer patient, you cannot expect your first oncologist to have all the answers concerning your tumor type. As a matter of fact, they often do not know the molecular/genetic makeup of your specific cancer or your tumor's particular microenvironment, nor do they know the tumor's response to a potential chemotherapy.

- Research becomes your job.

- If you can't do your own research, you need to get help. It's extremely important.

- There are numerous benefits to doing your own research, including truly understanding what you are up against and how to defeat it.

- Research means going beyond your initial pathological diagnosis and exploring the myriad of leading-edge research tools.

Lifelines/Action Steps

There are numerous ways to gather information about your tumor type. Here are some specific actions you can take to start your research process:

- Find information to help tailor your care. **Caris Laboratories** utilizes multiple technologies, such as next-generation sequencing (NGS), molecular profiling, and other cutting-edge tests to personalize your care. Caris has a website (www.carislifesciences.com) for both clinicians and patients, and it also supports www.mycancer.com, a new site for cancer patients that discusses personalized treatments.

- Learn the basics of cancer on the *Inside Cancer* website (www.insidecancer.org). This is a great, informational/educational website discussing the hallmarks of cancer, molecular pathways, and diagnosis and treatment.

- Find information about up-to-the-minute breaking scientific research on a variety of topics, including cancer, on *Science Daily*'s website (http://www.sciencedaily.com/news/health). It's updated daily with expert scientific data.

- Read *Customized Cancer Care* by Dr. Ralph Moss, *Outliving Cancer* by Dr. Robert Nagourney, and *Disease Prevention and Treatment* by **Life Extension Foundation**. These books contain up-to-date research and treatment options and advanced technologies that are not made available to many patients.

- Visit the website of Dr. Larry Weisenthal, MD, a renowned oncologist and researcher who performs chemosensitivity and chemoresistance assays on patients' tumors (**http://www.weisenthalcancer.com/Home.html**).

- Go to Ted Talks (http://www.ted.com) and search for Health Topics and "cancer." You'll find some great videos featuring cancer research.

- For mobile use, consider *Cancer.Net Mobile*, an application from the American Society of Clinical Oncology (http://itunes.com/apps/cancernetmobile). It puts up-to-date, accurate cancer information and interactive tools at the fingertips of people living with cancer, their families, and caregivers.

- Search YouTube.com for videos on your tumor type.

Summary

Take small steps every day toward educating yourself about your tumor type. It can make all the difference in your outcome. As overwhelming as it may seem at first, researching your diagnosis is a critical step in saving your own life. Time after time, I have watched countless individuals ignore this advice at their peril. I would not have survived had I not done extensive research. If you are too sick or too stressed to do so, use the tips provided in Chapter 3 to find a researcher and/or strategist. The knowledge you gain from this process will feed your ongoing Triad of Survival to keep you alive.

"You can rise above this.
There is a way through it.
You can survive."
— Mark Roby

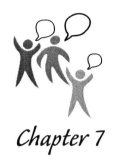

Chapter 7

Lifelines to Multiple Opinions

"All opinions are not equal, some are a very great deal more robust,
sophisticated, and well-supported in logic and argument than others."
— Douglas Adams, *The Salmon of Doubt*

It was late June of 2009, and I was on the brink. Over the previous few months I had collapsed a number of times and had to be transferred to various emergency rooms. Often I was short of breath, dizzy, and swelling up like a balloon. Furthermore, many of my lab values were going south, while my liver enzymes were rising.

As my liver began to fail, Kathleen and I made our way to a prestigious hospital in New York City. The major vessels in my liver were shutting down as the tumors grew. But my medical team could not pinpoint the exact location of the blockage in the vessels. They asked me to stay another week so they could find the problem. We were running out of funds and I was running out of time.

That night at the Hope Lodge (American Cancer Society), I cried out to God for help. I was guided to the Internet, where I found a renowned interventional radiologist named Dr. Riad Salem out of Northwestern Memorial Hospital in Chicago. Three days later I was on his operating table, where he spent two hours pinpointing the location of the blockage. After 10 days and two cutting-edge procedures, I left the hospital. These procedures made me stable enough to be vetted for a liver organ transplant.

I will never forget the care and compassion that I received from the clinicians and staff. Additionally, I am extremely grateful for the expertise of Dr. Salem and Northwestern Memorial.

Getting a Second or Third Opinion

Do you know what's really at stake by avoiding a second or third opinion early in your illness? The answer is your life and your survival. Cancer is an enigma that presents endless challenges to each and every oncologist around the world on a daily basis. If you are diagnosed with an advanced, rare, or aggressive malignancy, you cannot assume that the first oncologist you meet will know everything it will take to keep you alive.

What stops patients from getting second opinions? There are a multitude of reasons, including not wanting to offend their initial oncologist. Other reasons include extreme fear or panic, along with often being told that they must hurry into chemo, radiation, or surgery. What most patients don't understand is that they usually have a four- to five-week period following their diagnosis when they can safely explore these options. Of course, there are times patients shouldn't wait. These few exceptions include being critically ill or having a tumor that is causing a dangerous blockage.

A second opinion is an analysis or review of the diagnosis and treatment plan of the clinician who is treating your cancer by another physician or consultant. Hopefully, this would be a complete, thorough, and comprehensive examination of your original diagnosis and treatment plan that explores whether anything might have been missed, and looks at other treatment options that may be safer and more efficacious.

Many cancer patients would benefit from getting second or even third opinions. They include those who:

- Do not have an oncologist with experience in his/her specific type of cancer

- Have lymphomas, leukemias, and solid tumors

- Have been given death sentences or a grim prognosis

- Have been diagnosed with unusual cancers

- Are initially offered clinical trials (e.g., grim prognosis)

- Are offered major surgery right off the bat

- Are offered high-risk procedures, treatments, or chemo options

- Are seen at smaller or rural medical centers

The above list encompasses a lot more patients than most people realize. I personally have seen a number of patients with the above parameters not get multiple opinions or research their tumors and they paid the price with their lives.

A second or third opinion may turn out to be a critical lifeline for anyone who is diagnosed with cancer, and especially those patients facing advanced, un-usual, or aggressive malignancies. Consulting with one or more oncologists or cancer centers could very well tilt the balance toward your survival. It also may become an essential key to opening doors that you aren't aware of and lead to more advanced knowledge and treatment options that could potentially increase your survival time.

The benefits of getting multiple opinions are many. Consider the following:

- Having a fresh set of eyes review your medical records, initial diagnosis, and treatment plan, which could lead to a whole different outcome

- Reaching and connecting with top-notch clinicians who are renowned and respected within their peer group and, hopefully, your local oncologists can collaborate with experts in their field to give you the best care

- Possibly offering you more personalized, specific care for your type of tumor instead of the standard of care

- Possibly making you aware of new research or data

- Finding a doctor who might have more experience than your original oncologist with your type of tumor

- Leading you to safer, more effective treatment

- Offering you more cutting-edge, real-time research into your tumor

- Finding a doctor who is a better fit with your personality, while also offering you a way to see the whole situation differently

- Finding a doctor who is more open to shared decision-making than your original doctor

- Finding a doctor who might be better able to inspire hope and resolution for a dire prognosis

What if your oncologist wants you to get another opinion at his or her medical center? Be cautious: It's important to get an objective assessment and opinion about your condition and status. Occasionally your oncologist may have a colleague at their medical center who has more expertise in your tumor type, but often that's not the case.

When seeking additional opinions, you want to consider finding clinicians who are completely separate from each other and from their institutions. You want an independent, non-biased, fresh consultation; otherwise, you could be wasting your time. Unless you are in a major metropolis, and you are dealing with doctors at the opposite ends of town, I strongly advise you to go to a different city altogether when seeking another opinion.

Higher Levels of Expertise

Multiple opinions can help you find essential building blocks to keeping yourself alive. They are critical lifelines in building your contingency plans for your Triad of Survival. Getting opinions from sources that have a high level of expertise with your specific tumor type also contributes to better survival outcomes. Studies have shown that a significant percentage of cancer patients die from complications arising from their treatment.

While I was attending a conference on women's health in the summer of 2014, a cancer expert warned us to refer all patients with ovarian cancer to a gynecological oncologist with expertise in ovarian cancer. He told us that women's survival outcomes were much better after seeing this kind of specialist. He cited a recent study by the Society of Gynecologic Oncology in March 2013 which showed that 13,000 women with ovarian cancer were 30 percent less likely to die if they had guideline recommended treatment, yet two-thirds of ovarian cancer patients do not receive it. Often this is the result of being treated at hospitals that see a small number of ovarian cancer patients.

Part of my sojourn early on involved obtaining an opinion at MD Anderson Cancer Center in Houston, one of the top three cancer centers in the country. This is also the institution where I met the researcher who presented the concept to me of the Triad of Survival, which saved my life. One of their experts, Dr. Thomas Feeley, Vice President of Medical Operations at MD Anderson, was quoted in a *Wall Street Journal* article saying, "When you get cancer, the first thing you may want to do is jump to get treatment with the first person you talk to, but taking the time to get a second opinion about the diagnosis you have, in a careful evaluation of what treatments there are, can be lifesaving."[12]

As recently as 18 months ago, a young woman around age 50, who also happened to be an administrator of a medical clinic, came to see me for a consultation regarding an early-stage GIST (gastrointestinal stromal tumor), which is a complicated, potentially deadly cancer. She was on chemotherapy and doing well. Despite the treatment, her "performance status," or general health, was excellent. She agreed to go on a strict anticancer diet and was taking part in yoga and meditation.

Though in many ways she was a compliant patient, a couple of issues concerned me. She refused to get multiple opinions. She was being seen at a major cancer center and thought that would keep her safe. Even though I pleaded with her to engage other cancer centers and build her Triad of Survival, she refused.

Furthermore, I asked her to make researching her illness a priority. I even guided her toward books and websites specific to her needs to help empower her. Again, she turned me down, citing two things she thought took priority over my requests. The first was that doctors advised her to just "go on with your life" and "enjoy what time you have left." The second was that she didn't want to stop working full time until she retired 12 months later. Unfortunately, she died three months short of her retirement.

I was devastated that this fairly young woman and mother didn't know how to make survival her number one priority. I understand that she was overwhelmed, but that being said, I've seen this scenario play out time after time.

There's a lesson and a warning in this story. Most cancer patients cannot just "go on with their lives." As a matter of fact, patients facing a grim prognosis need to do the opposite: *They need to be engaged, find and secure lifelines, and demand personalized care. Not to do so may be fatal.*

---

12. Laura Landro, "What If the Doctor Is Wrong? Some Cancers, Asthma, Other Conditions Can Be Tricky to Diagnose, Leading to Incorrect Treatments," *Wall Street Journal*, January 17, 2012, The Informed Patient, http://www.wsj.com/articles/SB10001424052970203721704577159280778957336.

In his renowned book, *Anticancer: A New Way of Life*, the late Dr. David Servan-Schreiber speaks of the importance of multiple opinions:

> Patients are often surprised that the different physicians they consult can recommend such different treatments. But cancer takes such extraordinary different shapes that medicine strives to multiply the angles of attack. Faced with this complexity, each physician falls back on the approaches he or she has mastered best and has come to trust. As a result, physicians I know would never entrust themselves or a member of their family to the first advice that comes along; they would try to get the opinions of at least two or three colleagues.

I studied Dr. Servan-Schreiber's work at length and think he has written one of the best self-help books for cancer ever published.

This Has Never Been Done Before . . .

Multiple opinions may lead to better treatment options, or they may do the opposite and teach you about treatments that you don't want. During the summer of 2009, I was dying of liver failure. My clinical trial drug, Sutent®, had stopped working and the tumors in my liver were growing like weeds. I was running out of time, deathly ill, and desperate for answers. After two visits to Cleveland Clinic, the doctors told me they would vet me for a transplant. This is a six- to eight-week process of vetting to even see if you're a candidate. Then, if you are, you have to wait for a liver, which could take months or years. This was dicey, because thousands of people a year die waiting for a new liver.

In the midst of all this, I decided to visit a liver transplant center in Michigan to talk to the head of the department. During our discussion, the surgeon offered me a risky, major operation that had never been performed. "Mark, you're going to die soon unless something is done quickly," he stated. "I could relieve your tumor burden by taking out the majority of your liver, except for the caudate lobe. This has never been done before, but I think it's your only option."

He was sure that my liver would regenerate itself from the little tissue that was remaining in the caudate lobe. Livers do not typically regenerate if they are diseased and old. "Doctor," I said, "there are small tumors that I can see in the caudate lobe of my liver. Are you sure that my liver will grow back?" "Mark, you're up against the wall," he replied. "I honestly think and feel that your caudate lobe will regenerate and there might be some hope of survival."

I asked him to outline his plan at length and headed east for additional opinions from two prestigious medical centers. There, I laid out his plan to two of the most renowned liver transplant surgeons on the East Coast. They looked at the Michigan surgeon's plan and laughed. "You would never make it off the operating table," one of them said. They were both appalled that a surgeon would actually present this plan to a patient who was a medical professional, especially one that had fought for his life for the past seven years. That transplant surgeon took the cake for minimizing the risks of a potentially fatal operation.

Take Your Time in Making Any Big Treatment Decisions

Oftentimes, when you are sitting in front of yet another oncologist, you may be feeling enormous turmoil that can include fear, anxiety, or depression. You may even be experiencing brain fog or cognitive deficits because of exhaustion or information overload. What you don't want to do is make big decisions about going forward with a major treatment option until you have gone home, calmed down, cleared your mind, and researched it with your inner circle.

It's essential that you know the risks and benefits of the treatment plan put in front of you. It's in your best interest to step back, take your time, and research these plans carefully. I have had office visits in which the risks of my treatments were minimized and the benefits were overblown. I have also found that I am not alone in this experience.

Each of your consultations is part of your education process about your tumor and gives you a chance to develop more strategies and access more targeted, personalized treatments. It's a way to look at your diagnosis from every possible angle. It's a chance to find a clinician who specializes in your tumor type or subtype. Overall, it's a way to find suitable, specialized, less aggressive, less risky treatment plans or clinical trials.

When your back is up against the wall, my personal preference is to consult with eclectic oncologists who really think outside the box. Ideally, you want to take all of the knowledge and data you're gathering from each of these consultations, summarize it, and then use the best parts of it to build your Triad of Survival, but also so you can practice shared decision-making with your doctor. Choose those treatments that you and your team have researched thoroughly for accuracy and safety.

Asking the Right Questions

Before you ever visit a particular medical center or make an appointment with a specific doctor, it's a good idea to screen your candidates in advance and make the most efficient use of your precious time. Here are some questions you can ask to help you narrow down your potential medical center or doctor choices:

- Do you use molecular profiling at your institute? If not, where can I send my slides if I want a molecular profile?

- Do you happen to know if Dr. X is familiar with the molecular genetic makeup of my particular tumor type?

- How many patients has Dr. X seen with this specific tumor type over the last year? (If they don't know, ask for a ballpark. They should be able to find out.)

- How would you describe Dr. X's demeanor?

• Is Dr. X open to integrative medicine?

• Does Dr. X have access to or know of clinical trials for my type
  of tumor?

It's hard to say if you will be allowed to have a phone consult with the doctor
to ask these questions before making an appointment, but it would be well worth
your while to try. If not, you can try to speak with a nurse, a nurse practitioner, or
a physician assistant who works with the doctor you want to see to ask as many of
these questions ahead of time as possible. Doing this can potentially save you lots
of time and money in travel costs, as you are essentially vetting the doctor to see if
he or she meets your needs. Always be polite when asking these questions and be
sure to express your gratitude, because the staff does not typically answer these
kinds of questions.

Certain medical centers, such as Cleveland Clinic, offer online second opinions
for patients with cancer and other illnesses. The patient and their clinicians gather
data and scans, along with a summary of their current status, and forward it all to
a Cleveland Clinic specialist. The medical records and data are carefully analyzed
and discussed at length. A personalized treatment plan is then created and sent to
the patient and their clinician. This saves money, time, and stress. I have referred
patients on more than one occasion to Cleveland Clinic for this service with good
results.

You've done your due diligence and made appointments with several specialists.
Here are a few questions you can ask to help optimize your face-to-face visit with a
consulting doctor:

• Is there a chance I was misdiagnosed?

• Could there be any discrepancies on this pathology report?

- Since my diagnosis is rare (or unclear or vague), can you find out if the pathologist who prepared my report specializes in my type of tumor? (This is to help reduce the chance of misdiagnosis.) If she/he does not, can you please be sure to send my reports from your office to one who does?

- Do you use molecular profiling at your institute? If not, where can I send my slides if I want a molecular profile?

- Are you open to using off-label chemotherapies?

- Are you familiar with the molecular genetic makeup of this particular tumor?

- How many patients do you see with this specific tumor type per year?

- Would you be willing to have two or three of your patients (similar diagnosis) contact me to discuss their tumors and their experiences?

- Would you help me make up my own Triad of Survival? (You may need to explain what this is to the doctor.)

These questions can serve as part of your vetting process to determine if this doctor is the right one for you. After your visit, you can decide if this doctor is a good fit or not for your treatment. If the oncologist is telling you that molecular profiling, chemosensitivity assays, or animal surrogates will be of no use . . . be very cautious. Think twice before you go forward with this individual.

Getting the Most out of Each Visit to an Oncologist
In addition to asking the right questions, I can offer some other tips for maximizing your visits to your oncologist. Remember to do the following:

- Prioritize your needs into three major issues and address those first, in case you run out of time during your appointment.

- Bring someone trusted along to take notes or record the conversation, with the doctor's permission (always ask first).

- Go to your oncologist appointments armed with research in order to engage in shared decision-making.

- If you have the time to get all of your questions answered, take it! This is your survival we're talking about. No need to be shy. Ask the clinician for a complete written summary of each visit, including lab work and scan results. You can expect to walk out of the office with these in hand.

- Don't get pushed quickly into treatment; take your time to weigh your options. Use caution when making any big decisions on the spot in a doc's office.

- When you're feeling fearful, tell the doctor you need time to think about it. Get a second or third opinion in person or over the phone; do more research; use mindfulness (which will be explained further in Chapter 8) to get centered, calm, and ask for guidance; and talk to other survivors.

All of these tips are part of being an empowered patient who is prepared, alert, and ready for whatever might come up, even if it's bad news. Going forward, you need to lean on your inner circle, incorporate integrative medicine, and research the hell out of your illness. The more approaches, opinions, and lifelines you gather, the greater your chances of surviving.

Key Points

Multiple opinions are critical for patients facing a difficult prognosis. A second or third opinion should be made up of a thorough investigation of your original diagnosis and therapeutic plan by other clinicians independent of your initial oncologist and/or medical center. Furthermore, these opinions may lead to cutting-edge information about your case that could potentially be lifesaving. Don't make big decisions on the spot. Research shows that cancer centers and clinicians with expertise in your tumor type might possibly lead you to better outcomes. Multiple opinions may also help you to build your Triad of Survival, which could lead to safer, more efficacious treatments. Making lists and preparing questions are critical to getting the most out of these additional consultations.

Lifelines/Action Steps

Now that you understand the benefits of getting multiple opinions, here are the steps to follow:

- Make sure you have at least two volumes of *all of your medical records pertaining to your diagnosis,* one for you and one for your new consultants. This is critical.

- Do your homework and find two or three clinicians who have expertise in your tumor type (see Chapter 3 for ways to find a clinician).

- Prepare your questions carefully using the resources in your inner circle and discuss the results with them.

- Pick up the phone and talk to a nurse or physician assistant who works with the doctor and use the questions found in Chapter 6 on team building to see if you're a match.

• During your appointment, take notes and record the conversation so as to document a summary of the visit. Use the opportunity to gain as much information as you can about the nuances of your tumor type. Be careful not to make any snap decisions on the spot, give yourself plenty of time.

• Reference "Five Things You May Not Know about Second Opinions," from the *Harvard Health Letter* at http://www.health.harvard.edu/press_ releases/ five-things-you-may-not-know-about-second-opinions.

• Go to **Cancer Treatment Centers of America** for help in finding additional opinions. I have referred many patients over the past 12 years to a number of these centers, with positive results. As far as I know, this group of facilities represents the largest and most comprehensive system in the country that offers integrative oncology. Call 800-268-0786 to speak to a support staff person who will help or visit their website at http://www.cancercenter.com/.

• Consider an online second opinion, such as **Cleveland Clinic**'s online second opinion service at www.eclevelandclinic.org/myConsultHome.

• Go to *Consumer Reports*' webpage on health, doctors, and hospitals at http://www.consumerreports.org/cro/health/index.htm to help you choose medical providers; they have a rating system.

• Read *Second Opinions* by Jerome Groopman, MD (http://jeromegroopman.com/second-opinions.html).

Summary

Multiple opinions are an essential extension of your original diagnosis and treatment plan—especially if your disease is advanced, unusual, or aggressive. Don't be a passive/subservient/quiet patient who ends up being a statistic. The benefits of obtaining multiple opinions are many, including a fresh perspective and a more personalized treatment plan. Try and get a bigger picture of what is going on, and do not make snap decisions on the spot. Hopefully, these opinions will empower you to ask for personalized care, as discussed in the next chapter.

> *"You can rise above this.*
> *There is a way through it.*
> *You can survive."*
> — Mark Roby

Chapter 8

Lifelines to Personalized Care

"If it were not for the great variability among individuals,
medicine might well have been a science—not an art."
— Sir William Osler, Father of Modern Medicine

Aimee Jungman knew something was wrong. For several weeks she experienced stomach cramps, followed by sharp, stabbing, intermittent pain. While on vacation, she went to an emergency room. After a battery of tests, she was told she had a urinary tract infection and a small cyst on her ovary. She was prescribed medication and was told that the cyst would dissolve on its own. She writes about her experience with cancer in the article "My Cancer Journey," found on the Clearity Foundation website:

> What surprised me about the whole experience was that the clinical system seemed to dismiss my concern. As a woman who knows her own body, I was telling them something was wrong, but they told me that I was overreacting. They were incredibly nonchalant and explained that female bodies were always changing due to hormones or menopause, that it can be hard for women to accept aging, and that my physical problem was a psychological one.

However, the cramps were still persistent. When we got home, I made an appointment with my general practitioner, thinking perhaps I had an ulcer or some other stomach issue and would be referred to a gastroenterologist. I was diagnosed as having irritable bowel syndrome, but again, the diet changes and medicine did not alleviate the symptoms. I went for a followup to my ob/gyn where, with a transvaginal ultrasound, they found that the cyst had grown and scheduled me for a laparoscopy. They said it was a simple procedure—nothing to worry about.

Before the surgery, I spoke to several other women who also had cysts and needed the procedure. What concerned me was that my symptoms seemed more severe than theirs. Was I misdiagnosed again? I called my doctor to share my opinion, and it was on that call that I found out it wasn't a common cyst at all. I had advanced ovarian cancer that had spread throughout my abdomen to my pancreas, stomach, and liver in a little over two months. Because it had spread so rapidly and deeply, I started chemo the next day.

I was devastated and shocked. I couldn't believe that a woman who had been in the business of healthcare for 20 years, had earned an MBA from a top-tier school, and lived in a city with some of the best doctors in the world, could have this happen to her. Where was the transparency in the system to make decisions? Why wasn't the information available so that I could understand it and potentially act as my own advocate? How much experience did my caregivers actually have with the disease, and if they couldn't diagnose it, how were they going to treat it? If I couldn't navigate the system with all the education and experience I had, what would other women possibly be able to do?

The day after I was diagnosed, I was put on Taxol® and Paraplatin®, a treatment routine that has not changed substantially in 40 years, and although

I didn't know it at the time, wasn't going to work. My doctor gave credence to the stamp of FDA approval as proof that the drug would give me the best chance at a cure. *However, the reality is that most FDA-approved cancer drugs benefit only 20-25 percent of patients*—and in my case, the odds were worse . . . Even more frightening was that after the treatment failed, my doctor still had no clear insight to determine which chemotherapy would enable a cure. He had no insight into my tumor genetics, which left him unable to personalize my treatment in any way. For ovarian cancer today, if there is no response to the drug, physicians experiment with different agents in hopes that one will be effective. This "trial-and-error" approach is not only random and ineffective, but incredibly difficult for women experiencing the dramatic emotional and physical tolls chemo and after-chemo take on a body.

Personalized Care, Better Outcomes

Is personalized treatment included in today's standard of care concerning oncology? In certain types of cancer, such as breast and lung malignancies, the answer might be "yes" in certain circumstances, but frequently, I would say the answer is "no." The 580,000-plus adults and children who will die in the U.S. this year undergoing cancer treatment certainly wouldn't think so.

Not receiving personalized treatment not only could be hazardous to your health, it could even be fatal. Why is that? Because the current standard of care often does not include multiple opinions, molecular/genetic profiles, chemosensitivity assays, circulating tumor cells, or personalized vaccines. Moreover, it does not include integrative medicine, which could lead to safer, less toxic, and more effective care, especially concerning side effects.

The mission of this chapter is to help you, the patient, understand and gain access to safer, more personalized care. According to Springer, an international scientific and professional publisher (http://www.springerreference.com/docs/index.html), a definition for personalized cancer care is *the right treatment for each patient at the right dose and at the right time*. Personalized care is a customized approach using tumor research, integrative medicine/nutrition, and cutting-edge treatments to increase survival times. Such an approach is not generally known to the public, nor is it typically offered as the current standard of care, however, it is the wave of the future . . . and the future, for *you*, can be *now*. Personalized medicine is, therefore, an evolving model using specific treatments and therapies best suited to an individual's genotype and is driven by patient demand for safer and more effective medicines and therapies.

I am asking patients and clinicians alike to go against the grain and grab ahold of this transformational movement that is upon us. I will suggest that a significant percentage of cancer patients can benefit from this fairly new and innovative approach.

Most practitioners today would also agree that the term *personalized cancer care* includes molecular profiling that looks for a person's genetic fingerprint of their tumor. This means that a biopsy of a patient's tumor could contain genetic information that could potentially be used to reveal targets for newer therapies, which can be lifesaving. Moreover, a biopsy could also be sent out for a chemosensitivity assay. As Dr. Moss says in his book, *Customized Cancer Treatment*, when describing the use of this assay, "the effectiveness of drugs can be predicted and patients can be saved the time, expense, and adverse effects associated with the use of ineffective agents."

I would take this definition even further, suggesting that other factors, such as the degree of nutritional deficits, cachexia, immune deficiency, fatigue, and vitamin deficiencies, along with inflammation and angiogenesis, should all be ascertained and assessed before a personalized treatment plan goes into play. These issues are often underappreciated or ignored in many oncology offices and medical centers.

Many of the patients I have counseled have asked their clinicians for more personalized care, including molecular profiling, chemosensitivity assays, and integrative medicine. More often than not they were discouraged, turned down, and told that it wouldn't do any good, it's expensive, and not worth the effort. ***Don't believe it.*** Don't buy into their pessimism. Should this happen to you, contact me.

Research shows that newer modalities, such as molecular profiling and chemosensitivity assays, are beyond the training or experience of some oncologists. They have been carefully trained to only approve treatments and/or diagnostic approaches that are included in the standard of care. So don't be surprised if you don't get your doctor's approval right away. You may need to do your homework in order to persuade your doctor as to the benefits and efficacy of these modalities. But it is definitely worth your effort.

Again, it's imperative that you, the patient, become informed, use cutting-edge tools/lifelines, and personalize your care. Your life depends upon it. *We, as a country, need to start giving cancer patients every known lifesaving tool available.* These tools are currently available. The question is, Do we have the will to use them?

Your Cancer Is as Unique as Your Fingerprint

Many patients don't realize that the *secret to their survival lies in learning as much as they can about their tumor.* Today there are many technologies available for researching one's tumor. They include molecular profiling, chemosensitivity assays, next generation sequencing (NGS), and using animal surrogates as stand-ins for humans. These technologies may help a clinician assess their tumor's response or lack of response to many potentially lifesaving therapies. Unfortunately, a large percentage of patients are neither aware nor offered these options. This is very unfortunate, and I hope this book can help change the current landscape.

An accurate tissue and molecular/genetic diagnosis can mean the difference between life and death. A significant percentage of cancer patients today are diagnosed and treated by simple, histological modalities (originating in the mid-20th century) that are based on morphology (form of the tumor and cancer cell) and the organ of origin. What many patients don't understand is that each person's tumor is different and unique. Furthermore, tests such as molecular profiles, chemosensitivity assays, and TumorGrafts could unlock potentially lifesaving information to extend survival times.

TumorGrafts are portions of your tumor that are implanted in immunocompromised mice. After the tumors grow, the newer and older therapies are then tested for a resistant or a positive response. It's my opinion that thousands of lives could be saved by using the cutting-edge research that is available right now. *That is why many medical experts, researchers, and patients want the standard of care to change.*

We, as patients, must understand that each of our tumors has a unique genetic fingerprint, which could potentially guide your clinician towards safer, more effective treatments with better outcomes. Many recent studies prove this. There have been numerous news articles and academic papers discussing the transformation in the field of oncology. Medical professionals and cancer patients alike are calling for a change. They want to move away from focusing on the organ of origin in the initial diagnosis to using genetic profiling. Additionally, technologies such as chemosensitivity assays and personalized vaccines, along with animal surrogates, are leading to safer, more targeted therapies.

Dr. Stan Kaye is the head of the drug development unit at the Royal Marsden hospital in Sutton, England, and the chairman of the Institute of Cancer Research's section of medicine. Here is what Dr. Kaye has to say:

> We are genuinely moving from chemotherapy to much smarter treatments based on a better understanding of what causes cancer and what distinguishes cancer cells from normal cells.
>
> This knowledge is being turned into new treatments, often given as tablets that make people's tumors shrink, and it's just terrific. So in the next few years, there's going to be an increasing understanding that you don't treat

all people with a particular type of cancer the same way, and individualized treatments will increasingly take over.[13]

The article goes on to discuss a new research center called the Centre for Molecular Biology in England that will hopefully speed up the process of introducing personalized medicine into daily patient care:

> It links with Cancer Research's UK initiative to introduce "stratified medicine," where patients with cancer have their tissue sampled with state-of-the-art molecular techniques, to diagnose and target treatment . . . ending "lousy" cancer treatments for good.

Here in the United States, I personally have seen numerous patients benefit from the modalities discussed in this book, such as molecular profiles, chemosensitivity assays and anticancer nutrition. Cancer patients across the country would be ecstatic if these strategies would be included in the standard of care. Furthermore, I know these approaches would lead to safer, more effective therapies and longer survival times. With that in mind, let's get back to Aimee. When we last left her, she was in dire straits. Her story continues:

> This is where my journey took an amazing turn that most women's won't. A friend introduced me to Dr. Laura Shawver, a leading cancer researcher who funded Clearity, a nonprofit foundation dedicated to finding genetic cures for women's cancer. She ran a genetic profile of my tumor and recommended a revised course of treatment that took into consideration my BRCA1 and tumor specifics. Because I actually began

---

13. Simon Crompton, "A Simple Doctor's Quest to Improve on Today's Treatments," *Cancer World*, March/April, 2011, http://www.cancerworld.org/Articles/Issues/41/March-April-2011/masterpiece/460/A-simple-doctors-quest-to-improve-on-todays-treatments.html.

to understand why we were going down a particular treatment path and how that could change my outcome, I felt hopeful for the first time in over a year. I finally felt empowered and more in control of my fight. After surgery, I went onto a second course of treatment of Gemzar® and cisplatin, and was finally able to achieve remission after six months. I had a chance at life again.

Treating cancer with a one-size-fits-all approach is doomed to fail. As both a patient and patient advocate, I am appalled that diagnostic technologies are not routinely used to improve the likelihood of responses and, thus overall, patient care. No two cancers are the same, and patients need to know that there are often several choices of chemotherapy or drug combinations with different mechanisms of action for their particular cancer. This is especially true for cancer that recurs after primary treatment, when tests can be used to select and prioritize the drugs with the best chances of success. There are thousands of ovarian cancer patients who do not receive personalized diagnostic testing and, as a result, suffer toxic side effects without therapeutic benefit or die because they are treated with drugs that are not effective for their cancer type.

There are several examples of the successful use of genomic profiling in cancer treatment. The American Society of Clinical Oncology, for example, recently issued a provisional clinical opinion supporting testing in patients with lung cancer. The statement examined lung cancer clinical trials and found that when the cancer was treated with targeted therapies, patients had higher response rates, longer progression-free survival periods, less toxicity, improved system control, improved quality of life, and greater convenience [e.g., pills].

As you can see, personalized cancer care helped Aimee immensely and became lifesaving for her and others. She exemplifies the informed, engaged, assertive cancer patient. She also knew that personalized care involved shared decision-making. This is an opportunity to put your research into action. Doing so empowered her to go forward and increase her own survival time.

Common Biomarkers/Targets That Can Be Found in Tumors

Biomarkers are proteins, molecules, and gene mutations in each person's tumor that could be potential targets for newer therapeutic agents. Many experts have suggested that biomarkers have been significantly underutilized and can be potentially lifesaving.

Learning about potential targets inside of *your tumor* could be very beneficial in increasing your survival time. In order to save more lives, patients and clinicians alike need to get on board and carefully study the potential biomarkers of each person's tumor. I would not be alive today without a careful genetic review of the biopsy of my recurrent tumor. Furthermore, I suspect that the targeted therapy that I am on now (Rapamune®) could potentially increase the survival time of patients with other kinds of solid tumors. How do I know this? Because of my research and conversations with other cancer patients.

Patients with aggressive, advanced, or unusual malignancies especially need to get all of the information they can concerning their specific tumors. Often the current standard of care in solid tumors is guesswork, especially in the beginning stages. If your particular agent or agents do not work early on . . . you may be in big trouble. Molecular or genetic profiling is one of the smartest things you can do for yourself to start building your Triad of Survival.

Figure 3 shows a chart that describes some common cancers, their biomarkers, and targeted therapies. The first column represents the cancer organ of origin, where the cancer started. The second column indicates the biomarker, or the genetic aberration. The third column lists the FDA approved drug or chemotherapy. And the fourth column indicates the next possible step in diagnosis, which may be

Figure 3 – Molecular Profiling

Tumor Type	Biomarker(s)	FDA Approved Therapies	Technologies Indicated by FDA
Breast	HER2	Herceptin® (trastuzumab); Perjet®a (pertuzumab); Kadcyl®a (ado-trastuzumab emtansine; T-DM1); Tykerb® (lapatinib)	Fluorescent *in situ* hybridization (FISH), Immunohistochemistry (IHC)
	ER, PR	Faslodex® (fulvestrant); tamoxifen; letrozole; toremifene (ER); anatrozole; exemestane (ER)	IHC
Non-Small Cell Lung	ALK, ROS1	Xalkori® (crizotinib); Zykadia™ (ceritinib)	Fluorescent *in situ* hybridization (FISH)
	EGFR	Tarceva® (erlotinib); Gilotrif® (afatinib)	Sequencing
Colorectal	KRAS	Erbitux® (cetuximab); Vectibix® (panitumumab)	Sequencing
Melanoma	BRAF	Zelboraf® (vemurafenib); Tafinlar® (dabrafinib); Mekinist® (trametinib)	Sequencing
	cKIT	Gleevec® (imatinib)	Sequencing
Breast, Colon, Lung (non-small cell), Brain (glioblastoma), Head, and Neck	PTEN	Low expression associated with lack of response to Erbitux®(cetuximab), Iressa® (gefitinib), Herceptin® (trastuzumab), Vectibix® (panitumumab), Tarceva® (erlotinib)	
Lung, Ovarian	BRCA1	Platinol® (cisplatin)	
PEComa/Recurrent Angiomyolipoma/ Lymphangioleiomyo-matosis	PIK3CA, mTOR	Afinitor (everolimus)	
GIST, Desmoid, Giant Cell	KIT, PDGFRA	Gleevec (imatinib)	

Data is provided for informational purposes only and is not exhaustive.

Source: Caris Lifesciences and www.mycancer.com

a newer modality, such as the next generation of gene sequencing.

Let's take a look at ovarian cancer, for example, starting in the far left column. Moving right, you see the biomarker is BRCA1. The BRCA1 and BRCA2 genes are implicated in breast, ovarian, and other malignancies. In normal cells, these genes help prevent cancer . . . If you have inherited a mutated copy from a parent, there is a significant risk of developing breast, ovarian, and possibly other types of cancer.[14]

Moving further to the right, the chart shows the current FDA approved treatment, which is cisplatin. This drug can be given in a variety of ways. Sometimes certain women are resistant to this agent and are offered other agents, such as targeted drugs or agents that are currently in clinical trials.

When I had a recurrence of my sarcoma, I had a molecular profile done of my tumor and it came back positive for three targets: epidermal growth factor receptor (EGFR), mast cell growth factor receptor (c-kit) and P13K/AKT/mTOR pathway. The mTOR signaling pathway is an important and complex mechanism that influences cancer growth. It is overactive in a number of solid tumors.

Another Personalized Treatment Option

Another option for patients up against the wall is personalized vaccines. This research and technology has been going on for a number of years and is finally being developed for clinical application. These vaccines help mobilize your immune system to attack your specific tumors. The clinical trials that are currently ongoing have shown promise for a wide variety of tumors.

Northwest Biotherapeutics, a clinical stage biotechnology company, is developing personalized cancer vaccines based on a patient's individual biomarkers. The company has two versions of its DCVax® personalized dendritic-cell therapy in trials. DCVax-L is designed to treat operable, solid tumors. DCVax-Direct is intended to treat inoperable, solid tumors. The concept behind both of these therapies is to

14. American Cancer Society, September 25, 2014, http://www.cancer.org/cancer/breastcancer/detailedguide/breast-cancer-risk-factors.

mobilize the patient's immune system to treat their cancer. The patient's own immune cells and biomarkers from their tumor are supposed to "educate" the immune system to recognize and attack.

A patient's immune cells are first obtained through a blood draw. For operable tumors, the tumor biomarkers are obtained from a sample of the patient's own tumor tissue, which is collected at the time of surgery. For inoperable tumors, the immune cells are directly injected into the tumors in the patient's body, and the immune cells pick up the tumor biomarker target information in the tumor. Both procedures communicate the tumor biomarker target information to the rest of the patient's immune system, including T-cells, which in turn mobilizes the immune system to search out and attack any tumor cells in the patient's body that have the same biomarker targets.

So far, neither DCVax® therapies have had the serious adverse side effects that are seen with chemotherapies and some other types of immunotherapies. Most of the time, there are only temporary, flulike symptoms.

DCVax-L is in Phase III clinical trials for a lethal form of brain cancer called glioblastoma multiforme (GBM). A small trial of DCVax-L in ovarian cancer has also been completed, and a variety of cancer types have been treated with DCVax-L on a "compassionate use" basis (may be used on those who are very sick and have no other treatment options). DCVax-Direct is in Phase I/II trials and has been administered for more than seven different kinds of cancer, including sarcoma, pancreatic, colon, lung, and melanoma.

Experts and cancer survivors alike have been calling for safer, more effective agents for decades. I, personally, am very hopeful about companies like this that can quickly move from research to clinical use and benefit a variety of patients.

Becoming Your Own Advocate

From day one, when I got hit with the devastating news, I knew the only way I would survive would be to use an integrative, personalized approach. My situation was dire and the prognosis was grim. At the time of my diagnosis, there were only 125 other patients around the world registered in the Internet group HEARD, meaning they had the same type of cancer I was battling. Even though many patients in this group had a low-grade histological diagnosis, one by one they started dying off. Regardless of what I was being told by so-called experts, I did not plan on ending up a statistic.

Talking to many of my fellow survivors while on their death beds really motivated me to research my tumor type and find targets I could hit nutritionally and conventionally. I researched everything I could about rare sarcomas and their microenvironments. Ninety percent of my free time was spent learning how to attack inflammation, angiogenesis, and other targets. I always took my research to my oncology appointments so I could share it with my clinicians. I also had a number of phone consults around the U.S. and Europe that allowed me to gain a new perspective.

I was repeatedly rejected for liver transplants by numerous hospitals in the Midwest, however, as I stated before, my early research paid off. Liver transplant surgeon Dr. John Fung, whom I had reached out to starting in 2003, eventually became the head of his department and approved my lifesaving liver transplant in 2009. I originally found Dr. Fung in a clinical study of patients with my tumor type. I kept in contact with him annually and started visiting his office two years before my actual transplant.

One thing that impressed me about Dr. Fung was that he had coauthored some scientific articles regarding liver transplants and rare sarcomas. Moreover, Dr. Fung and his staff at Cleveland Clinic would always give me and my partner Kathleen excellent care, attention, and hope. He would go over each scan and test with us while discussing the risks and benefits of the potential transplant. *Not only that, Dr. Fung and the staff allowed me to talk to a number of liver transplant patients about their treatment experiences and outcomes. And you can ask for the same courtesy.*

Leading up to my transplant, I was increasingly short of breath, exhausted, and could hardly bend over because of the massive amounts of fluid in my abdomen due to my failing liver. I looked like a dead man walking, who was somehow six months' pregnant! My arms and legs were swelling up like balloons, and I knew I was on the edge.

On the morning of December 28, 2009, seven years to the day I was initially diagnosed with cancer in 2002, the transplant surgeons at Cleveland Clinic worked 13 hours to replace my tumor-infested, diseased liver with a new one. Many, many patients with sarcomas in general, or liver cancer, do not get offered such cutting-edge procedures. I am very grateful to Dr. Fung, my liver transplant surgeon and chairman of the Digestive Disease Institute, and Dr. Charles Miller, transplant surgeon and director of liver transplantation in the Transplantation Center, for vetting and offering me this transplant. I also thank Dr. Bijan Eghtesad and Dr. Christiano Quintini, who performed this miraculous procedure.

On the following day, I slowly awakened in the surgical intensive care unit. I could not speak because of a breathing tube, but I could hear Kathleen, my partner, and Steve and Theron, my buddies, standing around me trying to communicate with me. Seven years of turmoil, struggle, and living hell were culminated and turned around into victory because of the hard work of literally hundreds, perhaps thousands, of friends, family, and healthcare professionals around the country who helped me through those torturous years. It was at that moment that I truly believed in and bought into the four most powerful words in the Bible: "All things are possible."

Yet from that day forward, I was not satisfied with being complacent or thinking that my transplant was going to cure everything. In the back of my mind I knew, after communicating with other patients, that my cancer might return someday.

As a matter of fact, the tumor did eventually return in 2011 in my new liver. Kathleen and I journeyed to Boston and found a specialist who ordered a molecular profile on this new tumor. It was positive for an overexpression of the mTOR pathway, which is a very common target of various sarcomas and other solid tumors. I then sought out the best interventional radiologist that I could find in Michigan. That would be Dr. Scott Schwartz of Henry Ford Health System in metro Detroit. He performed a radiofrequency ablation, which got rid of the tumor, and subsequently my liver transplant team put me on an agent called Rapamune™ (an mTOR inhibitor), which is both an immunosuppressant and anticancer drug. I am grateful to Dr. Sheela Tejwani, my oncologist and colleague of Dr. Schwartz, for the excellent care since my transplant and keeping close watch on my liver.

The crucial point here is that cancer patients must use every tool available to make their bodies *cancer-unfriendly*. That's why all of us need to engage in integrative medicine, along with the tools described in this book.

What the Experts Say about Genes and Cancer

Each day, each week, cutting-edge, personalized cancer treatment discoveries are being made in the lab that could be potentially lifesaving. However, many of those discoveries never make it to the patient's bedside because of the lack of openness and transparency in the system. Many patients who could otherwise be helped are dying due to this gap between research and practice, and a number of clinicians, scientists, and experts are becoming increasingly frustrated.

In "New Cancer Biomarker Tests Stunted by 'Vicious Cycle,'" an article by Nick Mulcahy published in August 2013 on the Medscape website, Mulcahy discusses another type of personalized testing called biomarker testing, and why it's not been more widely adopted by oncologists today. Biomarkers are usually proteins found inside and outside of cancer cells and tumors that secrete substances or send out signals identifying specific malignancies. Tests to find biomarkers can be used to indicate whether a cancer patient is likely to benefit from a given treatment.

> Cancer biomarker test development and adoption has "lagged far behind" recent advances in cancer therapies, according to a commentary published in the July 31 issue of *Science Translation Medicine*. Despite prodigious advances in tumor biology research, few tumor biomarker tests have been adopted as standard clinical practice," write the authors, a blue-ribbon panel of representatives

from industry, academia and professional organizations led by Daniel Hayes, MD, clinical director of the breast oncology program at the University of Michigan Comprehensive Cancer Center in Ann Arbor.

. . . Without robust biomarker testing, the "promise of personalized medicine" in oncology is being jeopardized, according to the author.

Dr. Lauren Pecorino, a professor at the University of Greenwich, where she teaches cellular biology, also describes her frustration with the status quo. In her book, *Molecular Biology of Cancer*, she states:

The major flaw in the rationale of most conventional therapies is the lack of selectivity against tumor cells versus normal cells. As a result, the side effects of most therapies are very harsh, as mentioned above. There is a need to learn about the differences between normal and transformed cells at a molecular level in order to identify cancer-specific molecular targets . . .

In addition to the severe side effects that result, there are also practical problems with conventional therapies. Cancer cells, as part of a large tumor mass, will receive different doses of treatment depending on the location of individual cells within the mass. Cells deep within the tumor, and therefore furthest from the blood supply, will receive lower doses than cells on the surface of the tumor.

There is a larger context of cancer as a genetic disease. I would like cancer patients to have a basic understanding of how and why their tumors proliferate. Authors Vincent T. DeVita, Jr., MD, Theodore S. Lawrence, MD, PhD, and Steven A. Rosenberg, MD, discuss this in their book *Cancer Principles & Practice of Oncology: Primer of the Molecular Biology of Cancer*:

Cancer genes are broadly grouped into oncogenes and tumor suppressor genes. Using a classical analogy, oncogenes can be considered as the car accelerator, so that a mutation in an oncogene would be the equivalent of having the accelerator continuously pressed. Tumor suppressor genes, in contrast, act as brakes, so that when they are not mutated, they function to inhibit tumor rigenesis [the growth of tumors].

Successful cancer treatment, therefore, relies on identifying and then targeting the specific genetic mutations within oncogenes (also called proto-oncogenes in their healthy state) and suppressor genes. Cancer is a sophisticated, sly creature that can fool the wisest experts in the world. That is why many cancer patients cannot continue to be complacent and do what they're told without further consideration. If they want to survive, they need to drive their own care, find an eclectic inner circle, and research every possible aspect of their tumor. *It's time to stop telling patients that these concepts and modalities have no clinical relevance.* I was told this many times, but I did not believe it. In the end, this personalized approach saved my life and continues to prolong my survival time.

There are numerous advantages to receiving personalized cancer care. I will outline them here to benefit the patients who are not thriving under the current standard of care. According to an article in *U.S. News & World Report Health*, written in conjunction with Duke Medicine, specific advantages that personalized medicine may offer patients and clinicians include:

- The ability to make more informed medical decisions

- A higher probability of desired outcomes, thanks to better-targeted therapies

- Reduced probability of negative side effects

- A focus on prevention and prediction of disease, rather than reaction to it

• Earlier disease intervention than has been possible in the past

• Reduced healthcare costs[15]

I would ask each and every patient early on to work with their clinician towards personalized care. This does not mean using a cookie cutter approach of guesswork and trying drug after drug after drug. A personalized approach is looking at your tumor and finding out everything you can about it through many different avenues.

It also means looking at the whole person, including mind, body, and soul. It's about making your entire being less cancer-friendly.

Key Points

Personalized medicine is a relatively new model of healthcare that includes individualized testing and treatment options that offer optimal, targeted therapies for your specific tumor type at the right time. Such advanced tests/modalities include molecular profiling, chemosensitivity assays, personalized vaccines, and animal surrogates. Cancer patients, researchers, and clinicians who know about these options are up in arms because far too few clinicians tap into these resources. Personalized medicine also involves patient engagement and shared decision-making between patient and doctor. Doing your own in-depth research and getting multiple opinions are both great ways to move toward individualizing your care.

Lifelines/Action Steps

Cancer patients must demand advanced diagnostics and better, more targeted therapies that are safer and have fewer side effects. Become more engaged using the action steps below and work as a team with your doctor to increase your survival time.

---

[15] *U.S. News & World Report Health*, January 20, 2011, http://health.usnews.com/health-conditions/cancer/personalized-medicine/overview.

- Visit **http://www.mycancer.com**. This website, sponsored by Caris Lifesciences, discusses molecular profiling, personalized medicine, targeted treatment, chemotherapy, gene therapy, and immunotherapy. It also includes questions to ask your doctor.

- Learn about preserving tumor tissue at **http://www.storemytumor.com**. At the time of diagnosis, most patients are unaware that they can use their tumor to personalize their therapy. As their cancer advances, patients become more informed and discover that certain diagnostics and treatments require their tumor tissue be preserved, and in specific forms. Tumor tissue can only be preserved at the time of surgery.

- Visit the **Clearity Foundation** at http://www.clearityfoundation.org/ for lifelines for women, such as education about ovarian cancer, molecular profiles, and specific targeted therapies to increase survival times. The main feature is that it offers a "tumor blueprint" that provides information about key factors of your tumor at a molecular level.

- Go to **Foundation One** to get all-inclusive genomic testing services. According to their website (www.foundationone.com), "FoundationOne™ is the first pan-cancer, fully informative genomic profile designed to help oncologists expand their patients' treatment options." Use the resources in the chapter on Triad of Survival to collaborate with other patients to find more customized testing and treatment options.

- You can find out more about personalized cancer vaccines from **Northwest Biotherapeutics** at www.nwbio.com or by emailing them at patients@nwbio.com.

- Approach your doctor about **eviti** (http://www.eviti.com/), a website where he/she can explore your treatment options to determine which one may be best for you. Once your clinician enters your diagnosis and medical info into eviti | Advisor, your doctor will be able to compare the potential outcomes, side effects, and even costs of different protocols.

- Search the website **CureLauncher** (http://www.curelauncher.com) to find clinical trials that are a match for you, if needed.

Taking action on any one of these steps will lead you to being more empowered and engaged. The more the better!

Summary

The new world of cancer care is upon us. It involves leaving the old paradigm of the doctor as the preeminent authority to a more collaborative, team approach known as shared decision-making. Surveillance and testing of your tumor is critical, using the progressive tools described above. Don't forget, many of the secrets to your survival may be unlocked with extensive research of your tumor. These secrets may reveal potential targets that could be hit with safer, more effective treatments.

> *"You can rise above this.*
> *There is a way through it.*
> *You can survive."*
> — Mark Roby

Chapter 9

Lifelines to the Soul

" 'Come to the edge,' he said. They said, 'We are afraid.'
'Come to the edge,' he said. They came. He pushed them . . . and they flew."
— Guillaume Apollinaire

*I*t was late 2003 and I was living in Sutton's Bay, Michigan, a scenic tourist town just east of Traverse City. Someone had given me an article about a young woman who had been diagnosed with a rare sarcoma just a few years earlier. She was experiencing extreme fatigue and shortness of breath, along with pain on her right side. Following an extensive period of testing, her worst fears came true. She had a late-stage sarcoma throughout her liver and lungs. She was offered palliative chemotherapy and given three to six months to live. She sought out three more opinions and received the same grim prognosis.

Each day and each night, she cried out to God for help. She decided to change to a plant-based diet and spend her last days volunteering. The cancer was still advancing. While at a church service, a friend invited her to a seminar on integrative oncology. At first, she hesitated. She was so sick and hopeless. But she went anyways, met the physician, and became his patient over the next few months. They worked together using nutrition that attacked inflammation, along with yoga and guided imagery. Her family and friends also ministered to her using hands-on healing and prayer.

Twelve weeks went by, and she started feeling better. She gained weight, and slowly, her fatigue started to lift. She visited her oncologist and he ordered a scan. Forty-eight hours later, he called her with the results. He told her she was in total remission and cancer-free!

In many ways, her illness mirrored mine, except that I had to fight over a much longer period and use more conventional strategies that I continue to need.

The Cumulative Effects of Chronic Fear, Anxiety, and Stress

There is a multitude of ways to feed and nurture our souls. As cancer patients, we hear many voices telling us what to do, where to go, and how to feel. This chapter is about finding that one voice inside of you that can give you guidance and lead you to safety. Furthermore, this voice can help you to discern the most direct pathway to remission and freedom.

Cancer is actually a battle for our minds and souls, because our brains and nervous systems are critical drivers of our health. It is essential that patients understand the mind-body-spirit connection and its implications. Many people do not realize that there is a direct anatomical connection between our brain and our heart. Additionally, our heart is a conduit to our soul.

In our current state, there is an overload of information, technology, and data that sways us away from the concept of self-healing. The old adage "God helps those who help themselves" is true. Patients must understand that how they feel, what they think, and what they tell themselves directly influences their outcomes.

This chapter shares another critical lifeline that I turned to many times, and still do, to help me survive: **God**. Instead of listening to the multitude of chaotic voices coming at me when I was sick, I chose to surrender my fear and confusion to God. You can do the same. There are many different interpretations of the word "God" or the divine. Whatever meaning you attribute to this word is up to you. There are also many paths to spiritual awakening and finding your soul.

Please don't get caught up in terminology when reading this chapter. This is a very personal topic.

There has been a growing epidemic of stress, fear, and anger in the U.S. over the past 15 years. Many people do not even know what they are stressed or angry about, but they go "see their doctors" and ask for medication, including psychotropic drugs, to deal with their feelings. These same patients, along with their physicians, downplay or don't even acknowledge the cumulative effects of their unhealthy lifestyles and negative thoughts. They can and do lead to many physical and emotional symptoms that can push people over the edge.

During my daily rounds in the medical facilities, I have staff members, including physicians and nurses, come up to me privately to share the intimate details of their lives. Many of them have tremendous stressors that they typically don't talk about to other people. They suffer in silence. Moreover, a number of the patients I see are experiencing depression and anxiety secondary to their physical symptoms. Clinicians may not connect the dots between their patients' emotional and spiritual health and their physical health.

About 20 years ago, I read a study that made the connection between experiencing trauma, such as multiple divorces, losing children, and financial losses, and a diagnosis of terminal cancer. *Emotional and psychological stress has been scientifically proven to harm the immune system and cause significant inflammation that can set the stage for life-threatening illnesses such as cancer.*

The science of psychoneuroimmunology (PNI) is the study of the interaction between psychological processes and the nervous and immune systems of the human body. This field has been evolving over the past few decades in this country, but the research is often ignored or buried by many medical institutions in favor of exclusively conventional strategies. It's critical that patients understand the connection between their emotional, psychological, and physical health and their survival. And how we deal with emotional, psychological, and physical stress is often dependent upon our spiritual perceptions.

My mentor, Dr. Jerry Jampolsky, wrote the following in his renowned book, *Teach Only Love*:

> As we emerge from the birth canal, we enter the world desperately struggling for breath. Most of us travel through life continuing to struggle, feeling unloved and alone. All too often we are afraid: afraid of sickness and death, afraid of God, even afraid of continuing to live. Often we leave the same way we entered it—desperately struggling for breath.

And in the book *The Four Agreements*, Dr. Don Miguel Ruiz writes:

> If we look at human society, we see a place so difficult to live in because it is ruled by fear. Throughout the world, we see human suffering, anger, revenge, addictions, violence in the street, and tremendous injustice. We keep searching, when everything is already inside us. We don't see the truth because we are blind. What blinds us are all those false beliefs we have in our mind. We have the need to be right and to make others wrong. We trust what we believe, and our beliefs set us up for suffering.

> We cannot see who we truly are, we cannot see that we are not free. That is why humans resist life. To be alive is the biggest fear humans have.

There are a number of patients whom I have examined over the past three decades who told me they weren't even sure they had a soul. As a clinician, I have taken the histories of countless patients in various clinical settings. In the ER, I might have taken between 30-40 patient histories a day. Oftentimes, I would ask patients about their family situations or levels of stress. On an intermittent basis, a number of patients seemed perplexed and surprised. Occasionally, these patients would raise their voices, become agitated, and ask, "What do these questions have to do with my health?" Some would even get distraught and demand that I only concentrate on strictly "medical" issues. Sometimes I would even go further and ask if they had ever heard of the mind-body-spirit connection. Often the answer was "no."

Dr. Jampolsky provides another perspective on this connection. In his book, *Teach Only Love*, he states:

> I believe that there is another way of looking at life that makes it possible for us to walk through this world in love, at peace, and without fear. This other way requires no external battles, but only that we heal ourselves. It is a process that I call "attitudinal healing" because it is an internal and primarily mental process.
>
> . . . The mind can be retrained. Within this fact lies our freedom. No matter how often we have misused it, the mind can be utilized in a way that it is so positive that at first it is beyond anything we can imagine.

This process of attitudinal healing has been a critical lifeline in my survival. Moreover, I have talked to many of Dr. Jampolsky's cancer patients who were given no hope of survival. I was impressed that many of them, like myself, were still alive using these concepts. As a matter of fact, all of them, including myself, are grateful for his legacy. We are all testimonies to the concept that nothing is impossible, if we give ourselves and our lives over to God.

Is God Really Listening?

Lee Coit talks about learning to discern between our inside and outside voices in his book *Listening: How to increase Awareness of Your Inner Guide*:

> There is a power in us that is of God . . . This power is reached in a most unusual way—by "going inside" ourselves . . . We may reach it quite simply by just letting go of all the babble and churning within our minds—reaching below this noisy level to the peace and strength that constantly abides in us.

Don't underestimate the power of your thoughts and beliefs. They could actually save your life. Many patients don't understand how to move their thoughts away from their lower self (fear, ego, and pain) and into their higher self (love, inner peace, clarity, direction, healing). These feelings of love and comfort bring all of us to a safe place. Cancer patients, more than anyone, need to feel safe. It's imperative that you discipline yourself to do the inner work of practicing prayer, meditation, guided imagery, and so on, in order to feed your soul.

Though I believe in a personal God, there are many different paths or belief systems for you to choose. Some call this life force God, higher power, intelligence, chi, prana, etc. Whatever works for you is fine. I encourage you to hold on to something greater than yourself. This is a big reason why I survived.

Sooner or later, many of us are going to be hit with something for which there might not be an earthly answer. Many of us will be in denial and think, *"No way, it's not going to happen to me."* What are you going to do if you are told that you have a terminal illness? Who are you going to turn to when there are few or no options left? Do you actually think that a magic bullet or a pill is going to save you? Instead of looking to the world for answers, you might want to turn to God. He/She speaks to us in many ways.

If we are so caught up in fear and anguish, we might forget to listen. We are taught and conditioned to think that many things are impossible, including healing true mental illness, AIDS, and an aggressive or late-stage malignancy. Patients and clinicians must understand that there are many ways and avenues to heal cancer. The one-size-fits-all, cookie-cutter approach does not work for a large percentage of patients, including myself. Everyone needs to choose their own path.

From the first day that I received the shocking news of my diagnosis, I got on my knees and asked God and Jesus for help and guidance. During my prayers, I told God that I did not know where to turn. I told Him that I was scared and worried sick. Though I did not pray for a miracle (magic bullet), I did ask that He guide me to the help that I needed to survive. My soul needed counsel and safety. It was lost in chaos and turmoil.

It was then that God put His hand on my heart and centered me so that I would be open to His wisdom.

When I first got diagnosed with cancer, I looked at the word cancer with a capital "C" and thought of Goliath. Cancer was a giant, hungry for prey, and at that time, it scared the hell out of me. But day after day, week after week, I started to see it differently. I wanted to cut that huge capital "C" down to a little "c." I understood that gaining knowledge of my illness, along with God's wisdom, could help allay my fears around my survival. The more I gained insight into the nuances of my tumor type, the less afraid and worried I became.

Cancer is a battle for one's mind and soul. No matter how sick we are, or how dire our situation is, our job is to give our worries, concerns, and suffering over to God so that we may concentrate on survival. Many patients put God on the sideline and neglect researching their illness. Both of these are big mistakes, in my book.

God will stop at nothing to offer us healing at any time, if we are open to it. It might come in the form of animals, trees, herbs, mountains, nourishment from food, other people, movies, TV, the Internet, or even strangers. If you are open and can believe, "anything is possible," God will use anything imaginable to bring you healing. How do I know this? He/She did it for me. God kept me alive and fed my soul during many critical periods when I was facing death.

Finding Your Inner Guidance

Regardless of your belief system, when in the midst of fear and shock, it's imperative to step back from the human drama and ask for spiritual guidance. In *Listening: How to increase Awareness of Your Inner Guide*, Lee Coit describes three steps toward finding one's inner voice:

1 Realize that we cannot solve, or even identify, our problems with our "worldy" mind—the conscious mind that we often identify as being us.

2 We must know that we have the power within us to solve the problem, and that we can strengthen this belief to the point where we are willing to let go of our "worldy" efforts to find a solution and be guided only by our "inner voice.

3 We must take the final step: Do it. We must calm our conscious mind of all its busy worry, all its attempts to find a solution, and go within— beyond this noise—to the quiet and peace that is inside of us.

Fighting cancer is a battle for your mind and soul. You must be cognizant of this 24/7. When the waves of fear and panic hit, that's the time go inside and discipline yourself to find your inner voice.

When it comes down to survival, any negative messages from your friends or doctors don't matter. *What matters most is what you tell yourself.* Your thoughts and your words carry the power of life and death. After all, who is in charge of your body? Most people think it's their doctor. That is a dangerous assumption, because you are then giving your doctor all of the authority and power. You need to take back your power and find your inner voice that can lead you to safety.

After multiple opinions, the effect of my death sentence started to sink in. Even some of my colleagues and friends started to ask to me the inevitable: Was I ready to die? Many sleepless nights led to more fear and anxiety. As time went on, waves of panic overtook my body and mind, leading to feelings of hopelessness and despair. Most nights were spent experiencing night sweats and severe pain in my right side, along with fever and shaking. In addition to the horrible nightmares three to four nights a week, I would think to myself, *How can I get out of this trap? It seems like none of my clinicians want to help me. They won't even research my diagnosis. My savings are running out. Who's going to take care of me on my deathbed? Am I going to die alone in agony?*

How could any kind of guidance come in while my body and mind were wracked with pain and fear? How could I make any rational decisions after all of my clinicians had given up on me? How could I not buy into feeling like I was dying when my body told me I was?

It was early in my diagnosis, at the beginning of 2003, in the midst of this turmoil that a friend and I were traveling through Tennessee. We were on our way to MD Anderson in Texas for yet another opinion. I had not slept for days and was writhing in pain from the cancer. One afternoon, I looked up and noticed a huge flock of birds. Hundreds of them were flying in formation, traveling with us along the expressway. They seemed to be leading our vehicle. Miles ahead I could see the birds flying over a very large structure in the middle of the expressway. As we got closer, I could see a massive, silver cross over 200 feet tall. We pulled off the road into a wooded area. I got out and knelt down at the base of an old pine tree. I looked up at that cross and saw the sunlight reflecting off the top of it. Seven weeks of pent up emotions and pain flowed out of me as I wept and cried out. I felt a movement in my heart, and a voice telling me, "Be still, take my hand, and I will lead you to safety." At that moment, for the first time in seven weeks, *I felt a glimmer of peace and hope . . . That was a huge turning point for me.*

Even though my body felt like hell, God's grace helped calm the storm in my mind. For the next few weeks, the fear and panic dissipated enough so that I could find the discipline to focus on positive meditation and guided imagery that I had learned to help calm me down.

Becoming an Overcomer

Years ago, when I lived in New York City, I was a member of Norman Vincent Peale's church on Fifth Avenue. Dr. Peale is well known as the father of positive thinking. I still remember sitting there listening to him speak. One of his common sermon themes was about being an "overcomer." He would say things like, "Overcomers knock down roadblocks, they overcome opposition. When they are knocked down, they think of victory and come back, no matter what the circumstances are."

Dr. Peale talked about what a privilege it was to be around overcomers and to learn from them. He inspired me to be an overcomer. I listened to a recording of that sermon hundreds of times during my illness. Dr. Peale would often teach that God's spirit in us is more powerful than anything on this earth. He would share story after story about people overcoming what seemed like insurmountable odds.

One Sunday in 1983, I was meandering around Dr. Peale's bookstore when I came across a small paperback entitled *Love Is Letting Go of Fear* by Dr. Gerald Jampolsky, a renowned child psychiatrist out of the San Francisco, California area. I read his book, and much to my surprise saw that in many ways, it mirrored my own. A lot of his work was focused on helping young people and children with catastrophic illness. He had developed a body of work titled Attitudinal Healing, which stems from *A Course in Miracles* by Helen Schucman and William Thetford. According to Schucman, the course was inspired by the spirit of Jesus.

Jampolsky was one of the first to publicize and summarize the key points from *A Course in Miracles*. He took 12 short verses from the larger text to develop Attitudinal Healing, thereby making the teachings more accessible to the average reader. His teachings made a huge impression on me. Of all the verses from *A Course in Miracles*, the ones that were most useful to me were as follows:

- The essence of our being is love.

- Health is inner peace. Healing is letting go of fear.

- I am not a body. I am free. For I am still as God created me.

One verse that Dr. Jampolsky would repeat often during his programs was "the body is but a costume." This really made sense to me, that I am a *spirit*, not just a body. In addition to teaching me that I am more than my body, he also taught me that "anything is possible." He repeats this many times in his books and tells his patients the same.

In 1986 I contacted Dr. Jampolsky to ask for assistance with a friend who had been in an accident and was critically injured. Dr. Jampolsky's schedule was jammed, so I could not introduce the two of them, but he encouraged me to study *A Course in Miracles* and invited me to come out to California to learn these principles. That led me to attend my first week-long course on Attitudinal Healing in San Rafael, California, which then launched me on a 10-year, in-depth commitment to study and practice these principles.

In 1990, while I was at his workshop, Dr. Jampolsky asked me if I wanted to start an Attitudinal Healing Center in Michigan. I gladly took up the request and cofounded the Metro Detroit Center for Attitudinal Healing with Dr. Laurie Pappas, who is still a friend of mine. I spent about 80 percent of my free time over the next eight years developing our center, which became a gathering place for people who were seeking healing, both emotional and physical. This center helped at least 15,000 people, including people with cancer or AIDS. In 1998 I stepped down from a leadership role and became more of a consultant. The center is running today.

So even though I was a highly committed disciple of these teachings, and a medical professional, I still experienced the full range of human emotions when faced with my own catastrophic diagnosis. In fact, I still do today. That said, I held fast to these teachings during my darkest times, especially early on after my initial diagnosis. And yes, it made a huge difference. They gave me hope where there was none and continue to do so. I hope they do the same for you.

Many of us don't know that we have a choice when we are in the fire. We also don't realize how powerful our thoughts, images, and words are, and the impact they have on our health and well-being. *A Course in Miracles* says that a miracle happens when love comes in and changes our perception of what we're going through. During the many times when I was gravely ill, I asked God for inner peace and safety. I was led to go into my memories and re-experience images and feelings from my childhood. Here is an example of one of those memories that has been most useful in my healing and survival.

> In the 1950s, my parents would take my sisters and me to a magical place in northern Michigan called Grayling (a town named after a type of trout). Our family had a membership in a hunting and fishing club located in 2,000 acres of forest. We stayed at my grandparents' cabin, on a pristine body of water called Simpson's Lake. When I was around nine years old, I remember my parents allowing me to take our rowboat out to the middle of the lake and fish alone. I recall throwing out my anchor and looking at the forest that lined the shore. I would fish for hours, all the while watching cranes, hawks, and blue jays fly overhead. Often, I could see deer and other animals come out of the forest and down to the shore to lick at salt placed on the shoreline and drink from the lake. I could smell the scent of pine and musk in the air.

> Many times, I would pull up anchor, take off my shirt, and lie down in the bottom of the boat and let the wind carry the boat wherever it chose. I could feel the sun on my chest and a sense of peace as it warmed my entire being. Here I was, cradled inside a wonderful vessel while being pushed by God's own breath. I could feel a connection with Him in my soul and mind like I had never felt before.

So many times over the past 12 years of my illness, when I have been on the ropes, God has led me to safety through these images. I would take my hands, put them on the broken places on my body, and breathe in these images of healing, love, and natural beauty. When I did this, I felt a deep heat go into various parts of my body, saw colors and light come in through the top of my head, and felt a loving presence, all of which instilled a deep sense of safety within me. In addition, my pain dissipated significantly, my muscles relaxed and softened, and my heart rate and breathing slowed way down.

This level of deep relaxation helped strengthen my immune system and gave my body much needed rest. The physiological benefits were undeniable. I know I would not be alive today if I had not allowed my inner being to open up to and accept the healing available to me from such guided imagery.

The Concept of Giving and Receiving

As healing as guided imagery is, learning to listen to one's inner voice is just as important. As I continued to push myself toward remission, I realized that I would need to change many things about my life. My soul cried out for stillness and peace. In order to attain mental and spiritual clarity, I knew I would have to face my demons, including multiple malignant tumors that had spread throughout my body, a lifetime of workaholism, and codependency that had hurt myself and others.

I spent many nights praying and reading spiritual books, like *Love Is Letting Go of Fear, The Four Agreements*, and *Care of the Soul* by Thomas Moore. I also read *Listening* and *Listening Still* by Lee Coit. The passages in these books gave me hope, which fed my soul. They also helped give me a sense of inner peace, which my mind and body sorely needed.

During the time I was on interferon, I experienced dangerous side effects, which occasionally left me listless and hopeless. I felt like I was going into a dark, cold death spiral. I was so sick, I couldn't function or even think straight. I sought out and found a wonderful counselor at Gilda's Club, and he helped me through some of my darkest times. I felt like I was a ship without an anchor. He helped reconnect me with my own soul through meditation and imagery. He also reminded me that I had many things to live for when I felt hopeless.

I remember what it's like to be up against the wall. I recall what it's like to be right at the edge of that cliff. Furthermore, I've been close to death a number of times.

What I want to share with you is that no matter how sick you are, there is always hope. You can be a beacon of light to everyone. You can give of yourself in many ways, no matter what you are going through. Jerry Jampolsky taught me that no matter how

I felt, or how sick I was, *nothing is impossible*. He also taught me, through *A Course in Miracles*, that giving and receiving are the same energy, there is an energy exchange. This concept helped save my life and can save yours. When I was engaged in helping another person, or "giving," many of my symptoms and fears disappeared.

I have seen countless individuals come back from the brink of death using these concepts. They realized that no matter how they felt in the moment, they needed to take action. They knew that action equates with life.

In closing, here is my favorite prayer from *A Course in Miracles*:

> I am here only to be truly helpful.
> I am here to represent Him Who sent me.
> I do not have to worry about what to say or what to do,
> because He Who sent me will direct me.
> I am content to be wherever He wishes,
> knowing He goes there with me.
> I will be healed as I let Him teach me to heal.

Key Points

Your thoughts, words, and images are powerful, and you can use them to help heal yourself. You are more than your body, much more. There is a direct anatomical connection between your brain, your thoughts, and your health. You are also more than your feelings. When you are in the midst of fear and chaos, it is critical to get quiet and listen to your inner voice. This inner listening can help guide you to health, peace, and safety. We can turn our pain and suffering around by retraining our minds and hearts to have a whole new outlook, one that believes *nothing is impossible*.

Lifelines/Action Steps

Instead of seeing yourself as a victim, there are many ways in which you can draw on your spiritual energy to help heal your illness.

- When making important decisions, step back and listen to your inner guidance to help give you discernment. This can make the difference between life and death. You will know you have received guidance in your decision-making when you feel a sense of inner peace with your decision.

- Actively connect, commune, and meditate with nature. When walking, be sure to look up and out at something far away. Focus on that point and breathe in the energy around you. This will help clear your head and remind you of your place in the universe.

- Remember that "health is inner peace and healing is letting go of fear" (Attudinal Healing principle). Practicing this verse may help you to think more clearly and make better decisions.

- Read books, such as *Love is Letting Go of Fear* and *Teach Only Love* by Dr. Jerry Jampolsky; *The Four Agreements* by Miguel Ruiz, MD; and *Listening: How to Increase Awareness of Your Inner Guide* by Lee Coit.

- Watch inspirational videos on YouTube. Some of my personal favorites are those by Dr. Jerry Jampolsky, Joel Osteen, and Leo Buscaglia.

- Access inspirational websites. Here are some examples:

  ▪ www.ahinternational.org
    Attitudinal Healing International is an organization of 100 centers worldwide. Here you can find coaching, counselors, events, and more.

  ▪ www.jerryjampolsky.com
    Meet and learn more about Dr. Jerry Jampolsky and his wife, Dr. Diane Cirincione. They have founded and led the Attitudinal Healing movement over the last three decades and are gifted authors.

▪ www.joelosteen.com
Seven million viewers each week tune in to watch and be inspired by
Joel Osteen's messages. His ministry delivers "God's message of hope
and encouragement."

These action steps could become potential lifelines for you. They have helped me
enormously to make clear and safe decisions.

Summary

Most of us don't realize that we can play a critical role in healing ourselves. We
can walk through the turmoil, the pain, and the hopelessness and choose a path
to freedom. Protect yourself and do not listen to the death sentences. You are
not a statistic. You are more than your body. Follow your intuition. Access and
listen to your inner guidance before making important decisions. Always give
thanks and be grateful for each day of your life.

> *"You can rise above this.*
> *There is a way through it.*
> *You can survive."*
> — Mark Roby

Chapter 10

Lifelines to Engagement

"Sometimes even to live is an act of courage."
— Seneca

The term "patient engagement" is a popular buzzword used by cancer patients and advocates over the past decade or more. Becoming "engaged" means being connected or intertwined in your own healing process. This leads to more and more involvement towards driving your own care and outcome. It's a natural progression towards a full commitment.

My friend and fellow survivor, Tami Boehmer, exemplifies patient engagement. From the first day we met, I have been impressed with her courage, fortitude, and passion to march ahead, no matter what the circumstances. Not only is she a gifted writer, she is an intelligent, dogged researcher who has fought hard to save her own life and the lives of others. She has just finished her second book, entitled *Miracle Survivors: Beating the Odds of Incurable Cancer.* What follows is her personal story of survival, written here by Tami herself. Tami is currently in clinical trials and needs your prayers.

The Buck Stops Here
I remember reading a line in Bernie Siegel's wonderful book, *Love, Medicine, and Miracles.* He talked about how the patients he saw that did the best were

not the "good patients" who smiled and acquiesced to everything. The "exceptional cancer patients," as he called them, were the complainers; the ones who asked good questions, the ones, who frankly, were pains in the ass. They were the ones who made it, despite a terrible prognosis.

These patients Bernie describes are "self-reliant and seek solutions, rather than slip into depression. They interpret problems as redirections."

I read that book when I was going through treatment for stage II breast cancer back in February 2002. It opened my eyes so that I could do something to impact my survival. It was a start. I was 39 and our daughter was only three. My oncologist proclaimed my prognosis was excellent—no lymph node involvement and the surgeon had clear margins after a lumpectomy. I was treated aggressively with a toxic brew of Adriamycin, Cytoxan, and 5FU, followed by radiation. If cancer didn't come back after five years, I was practically home-free, or so I was told.

As my life started getting back to normal, I slipped back into old habits. I continued drinking diet sodas, eating sugar, and sweating the small stuff. I became stressed out after being laid off from a job I loved, then quickly went to new jobs that were very unhealthy. I lost sleep and serenity, and my family was impacted as well. It seemed I worried more about a gap in my résumé than taking care of me and my family.

Fast forward to February 2008. I was working as a public relations professional at a large teaching hospital. I was extremely busy and stressed out. In addition to my demanding, dysfunctional job, I was planning both my husband Mike's 50th and my daughter Chrissy's 9th birthday bashes.
I started to notice swelling in my right armpit. It would come and go, and it

started to concern me. I called my breast surgeon, who was one of those rare doctors who actually get on the phone with you. She dismissed it, saying it was probably hormonal. I breathed a sigh of relief and went back to my busy life. But the swelling continued. In time, it was not going down, and I started to get severe shooting pains down my arm. Amazingly, I allowed this to happen more than once before calling my surgeon again and demanding to go in and see her. It had been a long time since I read Bernie Siegel's book. I had been a complacent patient and, I believe, in a bit of denial.

Now I wanted answers. She sat me down with the results of the ultrasound and gave me one of the saddest looks you could imagine. My worst nightmare came true—after five years of being cancer-free, my cancer had come back with a vengeance. The tumor was very large, at nine centimeters in diameter.

The next step was a barrage of scans to see if the cancer had spread. Since I worked at a hospital, I could easily slip downstairs to the radiology department. I remember retrieving my results and sitting in my office, staring at my PET scan report. There were spots in lymph nodes in my chest and, most worrisome, my liver. It was stage IV breast cancer. There was no one else around, so I let myself fall apart. In a few hours, my husband Mike and I were sitting in my oncologist's office wondering how this could happen.

We decided to go to an oncologist at a very prestigious institution 2,000 miles away for a second opinion. We were expecting hope, maybe a clinical trial recommendation. Instead, she told me, "You could live two years or 20 years, but you will die of breast cancer."

Mike squeezed my hand as we both started to cry. I knew my prognosis was terrible, but actually hearing those words was devastating. What about

Chrissy? She was only in third grade and she needed me. It all seemed so unreal. Then this little seed of strength emerged as I responded, "I'm too stubborn to die."

When we were in the car, my grief turned into anger. "How does she know how long I have to live?" I said out loud. "She doesn't even know me!" At that moment, I affirmed I was going to prove her wrong.

In those years worrying about recurrence, I vowed to fight it with everything I had, if it ever returned. And thanks to influences like Bernie Siegel and literature on cancer, nutrition, and holistic living, I knew I needed more than medical treatment to get well.

Taking a Holistic Approach

I made some significant changes in my lifestyle. I left my stressful job and made exercise, prayer, visualization, and affirmations a daily routine. While I was waiting in the car to pick up Chrissy from school, or in line at the store, I would visualize my immune system melting the cancer cells away. As I drank water—and lots of it—I would see myself cleansing the residue of dead cancer cells out of my body. While taking a shower, I talked to my body, urging it to clear out the cancer and thanking it for its amazing work.

To learn how I could build my immune system, I consulted with a holistic physician and read books on holistic healing. I spent time purchasing organic produce and supplements with cancer-fighting properties. I even gave up sugar, which I loved, with the exception of really dark chocolate. I started using eco-friendly cleaners and natural shampoos and lotions.

I focused on serving others in my breast cancer support group, at church, and by delivering meals to elderly people in my neighborhood. Most of all,

I began to devote time to enriching all of my relationships, especially with my family, myself, and God.

But despite all of this, I began to slip into depression. I had too much time on my hands to think about cancer and the possibility of dying. Then I had an epiphany one day during a family vacation. I would begin searching for other people with incurable and terminal cancer who defied statistics and lived years beyond what any doctor predicted. I would then use my experience writing about success stories from my public relations job to write about these cancer patients. I desperately needed a purpose in life to make sense of what had happened to my body to inspire hope in myself and others. I wanted to demonstrate that anything was possible.

I began with a blog called "Miracle Survivors" and began interviewing men and women around the country for my book *From Incurable to Incredible*. The book features stories of cancer survivors who beat the odds of terminal diagnoses. I believe this was a turning point, which lifted me from depression into being a thriver and mentor to others.

All of these practices gave me a sense of power, knowing I was doing something concrete to support my healing. And it seemed to be working. Remarkably, my side effects were minimal and my tumors shrank with every scan, and after 10 months I was in remission.

But as happens often with metastatic breast cancer, the cancer came back. I decided I needed to be more of an active participant in my treatment plan. I suggested to my oncologist I get a hysterectomy, an option he had rejected several years previously (before I became metastatic), saying I was too young. This time he agreed, and again I was in remission, for almost a year.

I learned at each scan that my status could change at any time. Any metastatic survivor can relate to the term "scanxiety." One of the hardest parts for me was waiting for the doctor to open the door with the results. The shock and fear of learning my cancer had returned again caused me to temporarily lose my grip on my proactive role I'd been acquiring in my healthcare. My doctor suggested a chemo regimen and I started it right then and there. No questions asked.

Three months later, I learned the chemo hadn't worked. I was angry—always a motivating emotion for me. So I sought another opinion. A friend in the chemo suite recommended an oncologist in a nearby city, who was known as one of the most prominent breast cancer oncologists in the country. At the time, he was president of the American Association of Clinical Oncologists (ASCO). He had written many of the research papers oncologists like mine have read. And, unlike my oncologist, he focused only on breast cancer.

Luckily for me, my local doctor was very agreeable about working collaboratively with this breast cancer expert. In addition to having another person focused on my care, I began to alleviate my scanxiety by picking up and viewing my scan results before seeing the doctor. In this way, I didn't have to wait so long, and I had time to research and review treatment options so I could discuss them with my physician.

My consulting oncologist suggested aromatase inhibitors—more targeted, less toxic treatments for my hormone-receptive cancer. Each treatment kept things stable for a while, but I soon became resistant. I tried another chemo, an oral treatment called Xeloda®, which kept things stable for almost a year.

Looking for a Lifeline

Around this time, I was looking for a cancer strategist. Using LinkedIn, I became acquainted with Mark Roby. Like me, Mark had been through many twists and turns battling an "incurable" form of cancer. He needed some advice on writing and publishing his book, and I needed his personal and professional expertise to guide me.

I was getting frustrated, and honestly, a bit jaded by my experience with the medical community. Even though I was getting another oncologist involved, I still felt like not enough was being done. I was particularly concerned about the lesion in my liver. I wanted it removed, but both doctors did not see the point, since I had cancer in other areas of my body.

Mark told me about having at least three contingency plans, which he calls the *Triad of Survival*, in place at all times. He encouraged me to think outside of the box rather than simply listen to what doctors told me. This made sense to me and helped release me from the shock and feeling of powerlessness I felt when receiving bad news. Instead of just blindly accepting what the doctors recommended, I became the captain of my ship. My role was to make sure it wasn't sinking, even if I couldn't guarantee smooth sailing.

Ironically, it was a woman who is featured in my book who led me to my next lifeline. Nancy Hamm had primary liver cancer, but was not eligible for a transplant because of the location of her tumors. A targeted procedure called Selective Internal Radiation Therapy (SIRT), which injects microscopic radioactive beads into the tumor, shrank her lesions to the point she was able to have a liver transplant. She encouraged me to check into it. Both of my oncologists discouraged me. My superstar consulting oncologist told me, "It won't only not help you, it'll hurt you."

I went to a surgeon Nancy recommended and he tried to convince me to let him remove the liver lesion surgically. He told me the tumor would never come back. I was irritated because I had gone there to get a consultation about the radiation procedure. I went to another surgeon who balked at the idea.

Mark encouraged me to take time to weigh my options, do research, and become more health literate. He called this "adapt and respond." Nancy referred me to a great lady named Suzanne Lindley, who ran an organization called Beat Liver Tumors. Suzanne, a stage IV colon cancer survivor and amazing advocate, told me more about SIRT and other options. I had a lot to consider.

I could see why so many patients blindly follow what doctors tell them. Getting different opinions and researching treatments can be difficult and confusing. But I knew more than ever that it was up to me to find solutions to save my life.

When I reported the surgeon's proclamation—that he could get rid of my liver tumor forever—to my local oncologist, his jaw dropped. He finally agreed that the radiation procedure was the best "compromise."

In September 2010, I went to an interventional radiologist who performed the outpatient SIRT procedure. The therapy was a two-part procedure. The radiologist and his team first performed a mapping procedure to determine the exact location of and route to reach the tumor. Then I would return about a week later for the actual procedure, which involved a single delivery of 90yttrium microspheres into the hepatic artery. I recovered in a day or two. The tumor was eradicated and my liver has been clear ever since.

The other lifeline I had in my pocket was my diet and exercise regimen, but like my medical treatments, I needed another opinion. I questioned the approach my local alternative practitioner was recommending, as it seemed extreme and perhaps harmful to my treatments. He was trying to convince me to do bioidentical hormones, a scary prospect to me since I had estrogen/progesterone-fed cancer. He called me the "most noncompliant patient" he'd ever seen. I took that as a compliment.

I didn't trust that the alternative practitioner knew how the supplements he recommended interacted with my chemo. I'd ask my oncologists about supplements, and they didn't know anything about them either. At a conference on integrative and alternative cancer therapies, I had heard of an integrative oncologist in Chicago. I started going to his center and began a new supplement and nutrition regimen. They performed extensive blood work a nutritionist used to tailor and measure the success of supplements they prescribed. And I felt they had a better handle on interactions with chemo, since the director was an oncologist.

I became obsessed with my new diet. In addition to sugar and processed foods, I eliminated white flour, dairy, and all meat, with the exception of fish. It was easier than I thought, as I already had made changes, and it gave me a sense of empowerment.

Life Gets in the Way

On February 15, 2012, my brother Mitch suddenly passed away. I listened to my voicemail. It was my mom. I was busy and didn't pick up, but decided to answer after she called again. She was frantic, screaming. I thought Mitch was alive, I thought that she was panicking and the paramedics would revive him.

I rushed to the apartment they shared. The firemen were just leaving. A couple of them were laughing. I thought, *it was a false alarm, just as it has been with my mom in the past.* I remembered rushing her to the doctor when she only had a paper cut. But this . . . I walked in the door and the policeman was standing there. The first thing I saw was Mitch lying on the floor in the kitchen, a tattered blanket over him. It appeared he had a heart attack or a stroke. It didn't really matter. He was gone.

I was thrust into taking care of Mitch's arrangements and helping my mother. My health took a back seat as I tried to "fix" my mother's life after the loss of her caregiver. She was a mess, more than usual. Already in mental and physical ill health and dependent on prescription drugs, she was like a drowning person unable to help herself from dragging her "rescuer" down with her.

Once again, it became extremely apparent how emotions and stress can impact one's health. Up until this point, my cancer was behaving itself, for the most part. I'd have slight progressions or stable scans. The scan after my brother's death and funeral was different. The cancer had spread extensively to my peritoneal region and omentum (the lining that covers the abdominal organs). It was an unusual place for breast cancer to metastasize.

I suggested a biopsy to make sure it was still the same cancer. It was. My consulting oncologist recommended the chemo drug Halaven®. It didn't work. I decided to "fire" him. Although he was known as a "rock star" of oncologists, he seemed to give up on me. He told me I could try a few other treatments, but there was only about a 20 percent chance they would work. I answered, "Well that's depressing!" "Yes it is," was his response. I found another consulting oncologist at a nearby cancer center, thanks to a friend's recommendation.

I was extremely pissed off and scared, feeling like the oncologists were just throwing darts at chemo treatments and hoping they'd stick. That wasn't going to work for me. There had to be a better way.

Personalizing My Care

Mark Roby suggested I look into molecular profiling to determine what drug would work best for me. I started talking about it on Facebook. Rick Shapiro, a contact I met at the Annie Appleseed conference for complementary and alternative cancer therapies messaged me to tell me about a woman who'd had amazing success with chemosensitivity assays. They became my newest lifeline.

The process was expensive and extensive, but it made perfect sense to me. I'd had many friends who died from being bombarded with chemo after chemo regimen. It tore down their bodies, and worst of all, it didn't work. I was not going to be a science experiment! If I was going to have poison put in my body, there better be a chance it would work!

The process involved getting a sample of the solid tumor, with a biopsy that would immediately be sent to the lab in California. There, an ex vivo analysis would be performed, and the sample tested against several chemotherapy agents to determine which ones would cause the cancer cells to die. It would also show to which drugs the cancer was resistant. It seemed to be the personalized approach I'd been seeking.

I didn't anticipate the toll the biopsy would take on my body. Perhaps the surgeon had to dig deep into my abdomen, but I couldn't move. I was shocked that it was an outpatient procedure. I was in extreme pain and a friend had to come and take care of me. I developed a urinary tract infection and the antibiotics made me so nauseous I couldn't eat. I lost 10 pounds in two weeks.

The results came back showing three top regimens the test recommended. I was astounded when I learned my insurance company would not approve the first recommendation, carboplatin and Gemzar®, because it didn't fit their treatment guidelines. I decided I could not wait for the appeal process to get the first choice chemo, so I asked my doctor to start me on Cytoxan®, which was down the list. It worked, according to my PET scan results. Every lesion decreased in uptake, and this after only three treatments! Before this PET scan, I was very nervous because I'd been experiencing a little pain and pressure. I cried when I read the scan, because it was the best scan I had in years.

I now had another lifeline in place—getting approval for the first line of treatment. But it was not meant to be. After months of going through a frustrating and draining appeal process, I was denied. And after six months or so, the Cytoxan® stopped working.

My new consulting oncologist recommended I consider Phase I clinical trials. Again I was in "adapt and respond" mode. I did a lot of research but could not find a trial I qualified for, and his center didn't have one for me at the time. I remembered my first "rock star" consulting oncologist talking about a promising targeted drug that was in trial at the time, but had recently been approved. It was called Afinitor®, and combined with the aromatase inhibitor Aromasin®, it was being used successfully to treat hormone-receptive breast cancer that had become resistant to aromatase inhibitors. I decided that was the route for me and I started therapy.

I had a feeling of dread going into the next scan, as some dear friends of mine had bad results from that treatment. Not only was I heartbroken for them, I was scared for myself. I started noticing pains that weren't there. I started going down the path of thinking that maybe I was just resistant to all treatments. But I wasn't. The day after my 50th birthday, on April 29, 2013, I received my PET scan results. They were quite remarkable! Every lesion had decreased in both size and SUV uptake (how they measure treatment response on a PET scan) or disappeared. Even the underarm lump was half the size it had been in the previous scan and showed a SUV of zero!!

I continue to follow Mark's advice, constantly looking for lifelines to complete my Triad of Survival. I know this will keep me alive healthier and longer. My friend, Suzanne, aptly describes it as hitchhiking to the next treatment. I have my eye on another targeted drug for my type of cancer that has received breakthrough designation by the FDA and is on the final leg of its clinical trial. I am always on the lookout for what's new on the horizon, and I continue to do whatever I need to in order to take care of myself in body, mind, and spirit.

It hasn't been easy, but I've learned to be one of those pain-in-the-ass patients. I'm nice about it, don't get me wrong. But I know that no one has as big of an investment in keeping me alive and well than I do. I may not hold a medical degree, but I've learned a lot about breast cancer throughout my 11-year journey. And I know my body.

If you lead a corporation, you hire good people with expertise to do their jobs. But you're still the boss. That's how I try to look at my medical experience. I have the right to hire and fire doctors. If a doctor gives up and acts like he/she doesn't care, they're off my payroll. I will look for someone who won't give up on me and has new ideas. And I won't just listen to them and follow blindly. I'll do the research myself, consult with other people, and make an educated decision. The buck stops here, as they say.

My daughter is entering high school this coming school year, and I am optimistic that I'll be here to celebrate her graduation and throughout her college years. My husband Mike and I even talk about where we might live when we become empty nesters. I will keep grabbing for lifelines and do whatever it takes, because life is too precious to leave up to someone else.

You can read more of Tami's story at http://www.tamiboehmer.com/.

Key Points

Patient engagement first starts with setting your intention to stay alive, while at the same time finding family and friends to bring into your inner circle. Tami exemplifies patient engagement because she knows that she has to look ahead and always approach cautiously, if she wants to stay alive. She also knows that patients facing difficult malignancies often have to lean on more than one oncologist or medical center to survive. Miracle or spontaneous remissions are difficult to come by and often have to do with hard work and persistence.

Lifelines/Action Steps

Patients who are engaged and participate in their own care receive better treatment and at lower costs. Here are some websites that can help you get engaged in your own care:

- *Inspire* (www.inspire.com/) is a patient engagement network with more than 100 national patient organization partnerships and over 500,000 members. Its core principle is that patients and caregivers need a safe place to support and connect with one another. This is where patients can share and learn about their medical conditions and treatment, and get support. Patients and caregivers can interact with one another to share their health concerns, participate in discussions, and even blog.

- *Navigating Cancer* (https://www.navigatingcancer.com/survivors#organize) is a great site to keep you focused and on task with organizing your care. You can use the site to help you keep all of your medical information in one place by recording treatment details, setting reminders for appointments or medications, and recording information for your doctor. You can even receive summaries of your doctor visits.

- *Livestrong Foundation* (http://www.livestrong.org/) is a multidimensional site that provides a number of tools for patient engagement. You can connect with your own navigator, research your illness, and seek out individualized care. There is a plethora of tools to let your loved ones know how they can support you through your cancer journey, whether you need support, want to start a fundraiser, or just keep your family and friends connected.

Summary

Tami and I would both not be alive today had it not been for hard work on our part. Patient engagement is not about doing what you're told, being complacent, and thinking that an oncologist and medical center will keep you alive. Patients facing difficult malignancies often have to go above and beyond the "standard of care," roll up their sleeves, and think outside the box, if they want to survive. Exceptional cancer patients that stay alive are motivated and engaged in the process 24 hours a day, seven days a week.

> *"You can rise above this.*
> *There is a way through it.*
> *You can survive."*
> — Mark Roby

Chapter 11

Lifelines to Financial Support

"A journey of a thousand miles begins with a single step."
—Lao Tzu

It was February 2004 and I was sitting in the infusion suite at the Orange County Immune Institute in Huntington Beach, California with vitamin C coursing through my veins. I looked to my right and saw a woman who was about 40 years old receiving a similar treatment. We started talking and sharing stories. She was diagnosed with breast cancer about eight years earlier, went into remission, and recently had a recurrence. Her malignancy came back with a vengeance, moving into her lungs and liver. She wanted to build up her immune system in between conventional treatments. She had worked as an artist most of her life, but had to stop about 15 months prior when the cancer returned.

Her long, blonde hair wrapped around her shoulders and down her back. She had high cheekbones and big, blue eyes. Her long, slender fingers looked quite pale as she picked up her wheatgrass drink. I asked her where she was living and she pointed out the window behind us. "I'm living out of my car," she said with a sigh. My heart sank to the floor as I watched her close her eyes. "I couldn't pay my rent, so they booted me out about three months ago," she said. "I take showers in the stalls at the beach," she added.

Over the next few weeks of my time with her, she never whined, never complained, and never thought of herself as a victim. She became my teacher.

Even though I'd been in the medical field for many years, this woman made me think of the thousands—and perhaps hundreds of thousands—of patients who were facing her plight: homelessness and bankruptcy. I have seen countless individuals like this woman fall through the cracks over the 12$^1/_2$ years since I was diagnosed. Here we are, the wealthiest country in the world, allowing our parents, siblings, and children to fall by the wayside. Disability and Medicare are difficult to obtain once you are diagnosed with a serious illness. It could be many months or years before a newly diagnosed cancer patient gains access to this support.

The mission of this chapter is to enlighten you, your family, and your clinician about the financial lifelines available. Unless one is very wealthy, most cancer patients cannot afford to become complacent about the financial help they'll need to save their lives.

How Will I Pay the Bills?

Throughout my entire life I have been a saver, not a spender. I never had debt until I got hit in 2002 with cancer. Early on, I was shocked that I was billed for copays as much as $2,000 from a single scan, even with insurance. I was getting scanned every few months and have been for the past 12$^1/_2$ years. My financial strain exacerbated my already high level of anxiety and led to many sleepless nights, worrying about how I was going to pay my bills, particularly early on when I was too sick to work. Even while I am in remission, I still have some worries and sleepless nights around these concerns. I'm still learning to turn this over to God and be peaceful, no matter what is happening.

During the spring of 2004, I was trying to keep it together physically, emotionally, and financially. I had just learned that a targeted agent called Gleevec® had failed at stabilizing my tumors. My finances were running low due to my medical issues, but I did have a small amount of savings left, along with a modest 401(k).

My research had led me to an immune institute in California that had benefitted a fellow sarcoma patient whom I had read about. I felt strongly that this was the right move for me at the time, though it was going to be very costly; I had no idea how I was going to pay for it.

I put out the word to my circle of friends and networks, and the response I got from them was overwhelming. The Metro Detroit Center for Attitudinal Healing, along with the Fairy Godmother Foundation, helped pay for my travel and lodging and put me up at a residence near the ocean. Their contribution was over $7,000, and I will be forever indebted to these organizations for their generosity and grace.

I was blessed enough to spend four weeks in California. My medical insurance at the time picked up around half of the cost, but I was responsible for the rest. I used up my meager savings and a large percentage of my 401(k) to pay for the treatment, food, and other travel expenses. The trip was quite enlightening for me, as I got to meet a number of patients fighting for their lives—just as I was—and share notes.

I met a man there who was a bit younger than me. He was working part-time and getting a little financial support from his family and friends. I was also quite impressed with him because he was seeking out an integrative approach for his cancer while living in the basement of some friends. He had lost most of his material possessions, but he was still alive.

I witnessed courage like this from the West Coast to Texas, as well as Boston and New York City. During the month I spent at MD Anderson in Houston, I wanted to make myself useful, so I helped patients out of their cars and wheeled them to their appointed clinic in the hospital. I met a number of children with their parents. Many of the children were wearing masks and appeared thin, pale, and exhausted. I found out that those parents had taken out second mortgages or worked two or three jobs to get the money to keep their children alive. It was not a happy time. When I saw them and learned what they were going through, it had a profound effect upon me. That experience helped me to understand what is truly important in life.

At the time I collapsed after my run in 2002, I was an average, middle-aged man, who was working two jobs and paying off a mortgage. During the first 15 months after my diagnosis, I was too sick to work and went on disability. After I started to feel better, I began a part-time job in the late spring of 2004, and have been on and off disability since. If I had not pursued the personalized/integrative approach as outlined in this book, I wouldn't be here. Yes, integrative medical care and getting multiple opinions have increased my financial burden, but I am still around 12 years out.

I did a number of things to stay afloat financially. Over the past decade, when I had trouble paying my medical bills, I made monthly arrangements with the medical centers and also used my credit cards. Today, the vast majority of any extra finances go to pay off my debts, including my credit cards, paying for healthy foods and supplements, and continued medically necessary travel. I still live a frugal lifestyle.

Bankrupt from Cancer

When patients are diagnosed with cancer, they often have many questions about their therapy. A big question, however, that often goes unasked is, "How much is this going to cost?" They want to discuss this with their physicians, but seldom do. Research has shown that patients, insured or not, often delay care if they think they cannot afford it. For the other patients who cannot put off care, the financial impact can be catastrophic. In the article "Medical Bills Cause Most Bankruptcies," written by Tara Parker-Pope and published in the *New York Times* in June 2009, she stated that:

> Nearly two out of three bankruptcies stem from medical bills, and even people with health insurance face financial disaster if they experience a serious illness, a new study shows.

The study data [was] published in . . . *The American Journal of Medicine* . . . In 2007, medical problems contributed to 62.1 percent of all bankruptcies. Between 2001 and 2007, the proportion of all bankruptcies attributable to medical problems rose by about 50 percent.

"The U.S. healthcare financing system is broken, and not only for the poor and uninsured," the study authors wrote. "Middle-class families frequently collapse under the strain of a healthcare system that treats physical wounds, but often inflicts fiscal ones."

Healthcare authorities need to understand and address the emotional stress of the financial burden placed daily upon most cancer patients. Furthermore, many patients suffer in silence because these issues are often not brought up during their office visits.

In many cases, neither doctors nor patients talk about the costs of treatments during visits, despite the fact that this would be of great benefit to the patient. In the June 2013 article "Cancer Patients Want Cost Discussion, but Fear Initiating It," found on the website www.amednews.com, author Pamela Lewis Dolan writes:

The American Journal of Medicine published a report in 2009 showing that more than 60 percent of personal bankruptcies filed in 2007 were attributable to medical costs. Seventy percent of those who filed had health insurance . . . An earlier study from the December 2006 *Health Affairs* showed that over 10 percent of cancer patients have paid more than $18,585 in a year in out-of-pocket expenses, and 5 percent have costs that exceed $35,660. These amounts probably are much higher today. Adding to the financial burden, cancer patients often must stop working, and their families must cut back on their jobs to help take care of them.

Referring to the same *American Journal of Medicine* 2009 report, a CNN.com article by Theresa Tamkins in June 2009 adds that "Bankruptcies due to medical bills increased by nearly 50 percent in a six-year period, from 46 percent in 2001 to 62 percent in 2007, and most of those who filed for bankruptcy were middle-class, well-educated homeowners." These are ballpark figures for all illnesses, but cancer patients make up a significant percentage of these numbers.

According to another article, entitled "Cancer Patients More Likely to Go Bankrupt, But Few Ask about Cost of Care" by Debra Beaulieu, published on Fierce Practice Management's webpage in May 2013, " . . . a recent study published in *Health Affairs* is one of the first to look at the 'financial toxicity' of cancer care in particular. The findings: Patients diagnosed with cancer were 2.65 times more likely to go bankrupt than people without cancer."

Hesitating to Talk about the Cost of Healthcare

Most cancer patients are under enormous emotional, psychological, and financial stress. There is a multitude of reasons why they are afraid to approach their medical team concerning financial issues, with just one being that they feel doing so could compromise their care. Yet keep in mind that your doctor can be an advocate when it comes to your financial concerns. Beaulieu's Fierce Practice Management article goes on to quote Dr. Yousuf Zafar from Duke Cancer Institute on this topic:

> "Many said they didn't think their financial problems were bad enough to bring it up," says Zafar. "Many said they wanted the best care regardless of costs," adding that they may have been worried that doctors might cut corners on care after a cost discussion. Other patients reported they didn't think it was their doctor's role to think about costs, or that physicians couldn't influence the cost of their care anyway. However, Zafar noted that from his personal experience as a cancer specialist, doctors do have the

power to make treatment decisions, such as prescribing a pill versus an infusion, that makes little medical difference but could ease patients' financial burden considerably.

Other reasons for not speaking up include the emotional and psychological shock of a cancer diagnosis alone, which can play a role by leading to short-term cognitive deficits. In other words, patients don't even think about the costs when they finally get in to see their doctor.

Cancer patients need to understand that usually their medical team, along with the hospital social workers, will be more than happy to work with their financial limitations when considering treatments so that patients won't become bankrupt. Clearly, patients need to be more assertive in discussions with their oncologists and other medical team members when it comes to their finances. Even though the costs can seem astronomical, many patients would be surprised at the plethora of payment options and support available to them from medical centers and pharmaceutical companies.

And now for the "unlocked treasure" when it comes to financial assistance. There are numerous resources cancer patients can tap into to help with their financial burdens, but one of the most important resources is an *oncology social worker*. Since many patients are not aware that oncology social workers can play an essential role in helping them with the cost of their care, they don't ask for such assistance.

Your Financial Survival

How much is it going to cost to survive your cancer? Probably a lot. Besides the expense of treatment itself, there are a number of other financial variables that come into play. Just consider the following:

• Can you keep your job?

- How many assets do you and your family have?

- Will you need multiple opinions or clinical trials?

- Will you need advanced, cutting-edge treatments to stay alive?

- Do you have health insurance? If so, how much will it cover?

Because newly diagnosed cancer patients are in a state of shock, they often forget to ask themselves these important questions.

What about continuing to work during your illness? How to handle work when you're sick is a very intimate, complex decision that needs to be made on an individual basis. Some patients may be too sick to work, whereas others may be able to work on a full- or part-time basis. This is a very touchy subject, because certain employers might be more or less willing to help than others. There are also disability laws, such as the Family Leave Act and the Americans with Disabilities Act that come into play with these decisions. This is a time to gather the people you trust and develop some strategies. I encourage that you cautiously discuss your health situation with your employer. Most are more than willing to work around these issues.

If you want to work but don't have the strength to go to a nine-to-five job, you can ask your employer about restricted or sedentary work. You might also be able to work from home or make other special arrangements. You might even change jobs or think about working for yourself on the Internet.

You and your family must put out multiple calls for financial help shortly after you receive a cancer diagnosis. Furthermore, you need people to help with fundraising, because the costs could be astronomical, with each treatment running $8,000-$9,000 a session. Failing to get that help could be catastrophic.

How do I know? I've been there, and I'm still going through it. The costs for diagnostic tests and cancer treatments are skyrocketing with each minute that goes by. Even many middle- and upper middle-class individuals and their families can be wiped out financially in a short time.

When I received my cancer diagnosis in 2002, there were few agencies I could find to assist me. Over the past decade, that has changed, with a significant increase in agencies and individuals who are willing to help. For most of us, social security disability can be an option. Many other organizations, including Cancer Care out of New Jersey and the American Cancer Society, offer other types of support. For example, the American Cancer Society often will help cover expenses for medically necessary lodging related to travel.

Hundreds and hundreds of people I don't know and have never met contributed to my fundraisers to help me survive. Why wouldn't they do that for you? Here are sources for you to consider, if you need financial assistance:

- Your employer and coworkers

- Family and friends

- Organizations you belong to, such as churches, synagogues, temples, and community clubs

- Second mortgages/loans

- Social security/disability

- Crowdfunding, Kickstarter, and other fundraising websites

- Social media, including Facebook

- Fundraising sources, such as benefit concerts, dinners, and silent auctions

- GiveForward.com, which helps raise money for the people who matter most in your life (www.giveforward.com/)

- Lend-a-hand-society.org

- Credit cards

- Your own website

- Garage sales

- Selling items on eBay or Craigslist

- Cashing out stocks and IRAs

- Adopting a frugal lifestyle—for example, cutting out newspapers, gourmet coffee, movies in theaters, cable TV, travel for pleasure and vacations, eating out, buying new clothes (shop second-hand and start using coupons)

- State funding through a grant

- An advance on an inheritance

Financial survival depends upon a multitude of variables. Engaging in frank discussion about this with your family and inner circle is imperative. Also, possibly liquidating your assets (assuming you have some) and living more frugally can help enormously. I personally have done most of the things on this list to stay alive. You can, too.

What about getting money for integrative medicine and/or multiple opinions? Again, the more engaged and involved you are, the better your chances of finding the funds. You need to be just as proactive in researching out for financial support as you are in researching your illness and treatments. Work with your inner circle and others to come up with imaginative, unique ways to fund your care. My inner circle and colleagues were very creative and imaginative in finding strategies to fund my care. For example, they ran walkathons, had garage sales, and held silent auctions, to name a few. Where there is a will, there is a way.

Key Points

Many patients are reluctant to discuss the issue of funding their cancer care with their medical team or center. They must understand that a large percentage of clinicians and staff would be more than happy to advocate for them concerning financial arrangements. Furthermore, there are many more avenues and options available today to help patients pay for their medical care. Finally, if possible, work with your employer and benefits office to create alternative work options, such as working part-time, working from home, and/or making workplace accommodations. *YOU and/or a dedicated member of your inner circle need to immediately start researching everything you can about your financial survival. Don't wait!!!*

Lifelines/Action Steps

When any of us are diagnosed with cancer, one of the first questions we ask ourselves is How much will it cost to survive? Here are a number of ways to help fund your care:

- Locate and connect with your oncology social worker to start a plan for financial survival; they can work miracles. Don't stop there, however, that person is just one resource.

- Make a lifestyle change to be more frugal overall to help pay for your care.

- When traveling for multiple opinions or clinical trials, work with the medical center and the **American Cancer Society** to get free or reduced rates on accommodations. The American Cancer Society has Hope Lodges in many major cities (http://www.cancer.org/treatment/supportprogramsservices/hopelodge/). These are free hotels for cancer patients.

- Delegate someone in your inner circle to start fundraising. It is not too soon to begin! Having the extra income will give you options you might not otherwise have, some of which may save your life. Here are some excellent Internet fundraising websites to get you started:

  - *Cancer.Net* has a superb list of financial resources for your review (http://www.cancer.net/publications-and-resources/support-and-resource-links/general-cancer-organizations-and-resources/financial-resources).

  - *CancerCare* is an excellent organization founded in 1944 that offers many different kinds of support (http://www.cancercare.org/financial). This nonprofit organization helps cancer patients afford copayments for chemotherapy and other targeted drug treatments.

  - *National Comprehensive Cancer Network* (NCCN) can be reached by phone at 215-690-0300 or online (www.nccn.org) and you can ask to be directed to financial assistance.

  - *The Isaiah Alonso Foundation* provides grants to families that have children with cancer (http://www.isaiahalonsofoundation.org/page/home).

■ ***The Patient Advocate Foundation*** also offers a national state-by-state guide to financial resources (http://news.cancerconnect.com/wp-content/uploads/2010/09/stateguide.pdf).

• Crowdsourcing is defined as a method for obtaining funding for a project or venture through contributions from a large group of people, typically via the online community. You'd be surprised by how many projects can and do get funded, everything from films to charitable causes. Here are some specific crowdsourcing sites for cancer fundraising:

■ ***GiveForward*** is an online fundraising platform that has raised $33,850,012 for medical and other causes not limited to cancer (http://www.giveforward.com/).

■ ***Indiegogo*** is an interesting site (http://www.indiegogo.com/) where posting a project is free, but the site takes 4 percent of the money raised. To encourage users to set reasonable goals, the site imposes a 9 percent fee if a campaign falls short of the fundraising goal.

■ ***GoFundMe*** is a platform that allows people to raise money for events ranging from celebrations and graduations, to challenging circumstances like accidents and illnesses. Based in San Diego, California, it's one of the largest crowdfunding websites currently operating (http://www.gofundme.com/).

• The cost of travel can get expensive, depending on where you need to go for specialized treatment. Here are some resources that can help:

■ **AngelFlight.com** is a nonprofit that serves patients needing transportation to or from the heartland region (http://www.angelflight.com/).

- **Corporate Angel Network** allows cancer patients to fly free on empty seats on corporate jets (http://www.corpangelnetwork.org/).

- **Air Charity Network** is a charitable aviation network that matches people in need with "free" flights and other travel resources (http://www.aircharitynetwork.org/).

- **National Patient Travel Center** (NPTC) connects cancer patients to available flight resources and may be the best place to start when searching for free flights (http://www.patienttravel.org/). There is no charge for this referral service.

- **Cancer Support Community** has a lengthy list of organizations that will help you find free flights (http://www.cancersupportcommunity.org). Call 1-888-793-9355 and a CSC Call Counselor will assist you in finding the right one.

Summary

As a cancer patient, you must consistently look for and use creative ways to increase your income and save money. Often people ask cancer patients, "What can I do to help?" Helping you locate the financial resources you need is a very concrete step and an invaluable gift. The more funding you have to explore options, the more secure you will feel. Adequate financial resources could be key to getting you higher-tier integrative cancer care. And your life depends upon it.

> *"You can rise above this.*
> *There is a way through it.*
> *You can survive."*
> — Mark Roby

Conclusion

*N*ow that you have read this book, my sincere hope is that you are armed and ready to vanquish the dreaded foe of cancer and not lose everything you hold dear in the process. *Lifelines to Cancer Survival* is about *patient power*. Instead of being a quiet, subservient patient, I am hoping that you will adapt and respond by using the strategies found in *Lifelines*, such as team building, multiple opinions, research, the Triad of Survival, and the wisdom of anticancer nutrition. Early on in your diagnosis, it is essential that you demand personalized care. Again, I ask you to discern between the noises in your head and the true guidance that comes from your heart. You do not want to let fear lead you to risky decision-making.

I have personally used about 90 percent of what's written in this book, and I'm still alive and kicking, helping others to survive cancer. Currently when I am not seeing patients, I study integrative medicine and also work with cancer survivors, along with medical facilities, teaching them this new paradigm of *Lifelines*. Even in the face of being seriously ill, my faith in God has led me towards additional options and strategies.

The more lifelines I sought out and grabbed onto, the better my chances of survival. Quite often, following one lifeline lead me to another, and another, and another. So walking through the chaos and the fear to take action often opened doors I never would have imagined. I believe God allowed me to live for a reason.

I had to work hard to beat cancer. And if I can do it, so can you. Hopefully, using these strategies will extend your life, and you will have an outcome similar to mine. Even though you may be facing enormous odds, you can fight back as I did, and survive. It is YOU who must stack the deck early on and make the cards fall in your favor. Successful survivors create their own luck as they go along, and are very careful about to whom they listen. They think and then act, often outside the box, always looking for new and unusual strategies and options. And they keep telling themselves:

""You can rise above this.
There is a way through it.
You can survive."
     — Mark Roby

About the Author

Mark Roby's fascination with nature, health, and science started at a young age. His grandfather taught him about nature, animal, and plant habitat, natural foods, and supplements. Working as a lab assistant and volunteering at an inner city hospital emergency room while in college, Roby became intrigued with the practice of medicine. He became a Physician Assistant, graduating with honors, and later obtained an advanced diploma in Naturopathy.

It was while living in New York in 1986 that Roby read some of the works of Dr. Gerald Jampolsky, renowned psychiatrist and founder of The Center for Attitudinal Healing, which had a profound influence on him. Later, Roby and Jampolsky became friends. And in 1991, Roby cofounded the Metro Detroit Center for Attitudinal Healing with Dr. Laurie Pappas. He was the executive director from 1991 to 1998.

Diagnosed in 2002 with one of the rarest, advanced sarcomas in the world, Roby knew he was up against the wall after clinicians from around the country predicted a short lifespan and offered only palliative chemotherapy. Besides radically changing his diet, he knew he would have to go way beyond the standard of care, if he wanted to survive. Roby became an incessant researcher, looking for advanced and novel testing of his tumor, and searching for eclectic clinicians who could offer him cutting-edge therapies.

A researcher from MD Anderson Cancer Center in Houston became his guide and ally, mentoring him with crucial strategies that are still keeping him alive. He has also had consults with hospitals in both the U.S. and Europe. Along the way, Roby had a liver transplant. Based on the genetic profiles of his tumors, today he is taking an advanced agent to maintain his remission.

For the past three decades, Roby has held clinical positions at teaching hospitals, which includes Montefiore Medical Center (Albert Einstein College of Medicine, New York, New York) and Henry Ford Medical Center (Wayne State University School of Medicine, Detroit, Michigan). Over the last eight years, he has served as an integrative clinician and consultant.

Roby has lectured extensively for over 20 years on Attitudinal Healing and integrative medicine. He is an active member of The Academy of Integrative Health and Medicine, and he's on the Board of The Emerald Heart Cancer Foundation, which supports women seeking integrative medicine.

Roby's story has appeared in the *New York Daily News*, *The Detroit News*, and Tami Boehmer's new book *Miracle Survivors: Beating the Odds of Incurable Cancer*. He is available for speaking engagements and consultations and can be contacted through his website (www.LifelinestoCancerSurvival.com).

Bibliography

American Cancer Society. January 16, 2013.
  http://www.cancer.org/treatment/treatmentsandsideeffects/complementaryandal-
  ternativemedicine/mindbodyandspirit/support-groups-cam.

American Cancer Society. Cancer Facts & Figures, 2015.
  http://www.cancer.org/acs/groups/content/@editorial/documents/document/acsp
  c-044552.pdf.

American Cancer Society. Cancer Facts & Figures, 2014.
  http://www.cancer.org/acs/groups/content/@research/documents/webcontent/acs
  pc-042151.pdf.

American Institute for Cancer Research. "Berries: Sweetening Cancer Prevention."
  ScienceNow, 41 Summer 2012.
  http://www.aicr.org/assets/docs/pdf/sciencenow/sciencenow-41.pdf.

American Society of Clinical Oncology. "The State of Cancer Care in America, 2014: A
  Report by The American Society of Clinical Oncology." *Journal of Oncology Practice*,
  March 10, 2014. http://jop.ascopubs.org/content/early/2014/03/10/JOP.2014.001386.

Bakalar, Nicholas. "Risks: More Red Meat, More Mortality." *New York Times*,
  March 12, 2012. http://www.nytimes.com/2012/03/13/health/research/red-meat-
  linked-to-cancer-and-heart-disease.html?_r=0.

Barnard, Neal D., MD. *Foods Can Save Your Life: Leading Experts Tell You Why.*
  McKinney, TX: The Magni Company, 1996.

Block, Keith I., MD. *Life over Cancer: The Block Center Program for Integrative
  Cancer Treatment.* New York: Bantam Dell, 2009.

Boehmer, Tami. *From Incurable to Incredible.* CreateSpace, 2010.

Boehmer, Tami. *Miracle Survivors* website. http://www.tamiboehmer.com/.

Campbell, T. Colin, PhD, and Thomas M. Campbell II, MD. *The China Study: The Most Comprehensive Study of Nutrition Ever Conducted and the Startling Implications for Diet, Weight Loss, and Long-Term Health.* Dallas: BenBella Books, 2006.

CANCERactive. "Red Meat, Cows' Dairy and Cancer – Red Meat, Inflammation and Cancer Risk." CANCERactive, October 3, 2010. http://www.canceractive.com/cancer-active-page-link.aspx?=2135&Title=Red%20Meat,%20Cows%27%20Dairy%20and%20cancer.

Coit, Lee. *Listening: How to Increase Awareness of Your Inner Guide.* Carlsbad, CA: Hay House, 1996.

Coit, Lee. *Listening . . . Still: How to Increase Your Acceptance of Perfection.* Carlsbad, CA: Hay House, 1994.

Crompton, Simon. "A Simple Doctor's Quest to Improve on Today's Treatments." *Cancer World,* March/April, 2011. http://www.cancerworld.org/Articles/Issues/41/March-April-2011/masterpiece/460/A-simple-doctors-quest-to-improve-on-todays-treatments.html.

DeVita, Vincent T., Jr., MD, Theodore S. Lawrence, MD, PhD, and Steven A. Rosenberg, MD, Eds. *Cancer Principles & Practice of Oncology: Primer of the Molecular Biology of Cancer.* Philadelphia: Lippincott Willams & Wilkens, 2011.

http://www.doctoroz.com/article/5-foods-starve-cancer.

FoodforBreastCancer.com. "High Glycemic Load Diet Increases Risk of Breast Cancer." FoodforBreastCancer.com. http://foodforbreastcancer.com/articles/high-glycemic-load-diet-increases-risk-of-breast-cancer.

Frähm, Anne E. and David J Frähm. *A Cancer Battle Plan.* New York: Tarcher, 1997.

Frankel, Moshe, MD. www.moshefrenkelmd.com.

Gray, Nathan. "Flavonoid-rich Diet May Reduce Risk of Type II Diabetes: Study."
    Nutraingredients.com, January 20, 2014. http://www.nutraingredients.com/Re-
    search/Flavonoid-rich-diet-may-reduce-risk-of-type-2-diabetes-Study.

H. Lee Moffitt Cancer Center & Research Institute. "Acidic Microenvironment in
    Tumors Aid Tumor Cell Survival, Researchers Find." *Science Daily*, www.sci-
    encedaily.com, September 6, 2012.
    http://www.sciencedaily.com/releases/2012/09/120906074249.htm.

Hanahan, Douglas and Robert Weinberg. "The Hallmarks of Cancer." *Cell,* January 2000.

Himmelstein, David U., MD, Deborah Thorne, PhD, Elizabeth Warren, JD, and Steffie
    Woolhandler, MD, MPH. "Medical Bankruptcy in the United States, 2007: Re-
    sults of a National Study." *The American Journal of Medicine,* August 2009,
    Volume 122, Issue 8. http://www.amjmed.com/article/S0002-
    9343%2809%2900404-5/abstract.

Hu, J., C. La Vecchia, L.S. Augustin, E. Negri, M. de Groh, H. Morrison, and L. Mery,
    The Canadian Cancer Registries Epidemiology Research Group. "Glycemic
    Index, Glycemic Load and Cancer Risk." *Annals of Oncology*, July 25, 2012.
    http://annonc.oxfordjournals.org/content/24/1/245.full.

Jampolsky, Gerald G., MD. *Teach Only Love: The Twelve Principles of Attitudinal
    Healing*. New York: Bantam, 1984.

Jampolsky, Gerald G., MD. *Love Is Letting Go of Fear.* New York: Celestial Arts, 1979.

Jungman, Aimee. "My Cancer Journey." Clearity Foundation.
    http://www.clearityfoundation.org/pdf/dm_16_my_cancer_journey_single.pdf.

Kain, Debra. "How Eating Red Meat Can Spur Cancer Progression." UC San Diego
        News Center, November 13, 2008.
        http://ucsdnews.ucsd.edu/archive/newsrel/health/11-08RedMeatCancer.asp.

Landro, Laura. "What If the Doctor Is Wrong? Some Cancers, Asthma, Other Conditions
        Can Be Tricky to Diagnose, Leading to Incorrect Treatments." The Informed
        Patient, *Wall Street Journal*, January 17, 2012.
        http://www.wsj.com/articles/SB10001424052970203721704577159280778957336.

Leaf, Clifton. *The Truth in Small Doses: Why We Are Losing the War on Cancer and
        How to Win It.* New York: Simon & Schuster, 2013.

Lewis Dolan, Pamela. "Cancer Patients Want Cost Discussion, but Fear Initiating It."
        Amednews.com, June 10, 2013.
        http://www.amednews.com/article/20130610/business/130619990/4/.

Madrimasd. "Excess Sugar Linked to Cancer." *Science Daily*, February 1, 2013.
        http://www.sciencedaily.com/releases/2013/02/130201100149.htm.

Middelmann-Whitney, Conner. *Zest for Life: The Mediterranean Anti-Cancer Diet.*
        Honeybourne Publishing, 2011.

Moore, Thomas. *Care of the Soul: A Guide for Cultivating Depth and Sacredness in
        Everyday Life.* New York: HarperCollins, 1992.

Moss, Ralph, PhD. *Customized Cancer Treatment.* NY: Equinox Press, 2010.

Mukherjee, Siddhartha. *The Emperor of All Maladies: The Biography of Cancer.* New
        York: Scribner, 2010.

Mulcahy, Nick. "New Cancer Biomarker Tests Stunted by 'Vicious Cycle.'"
        Medscape.com, August 5, 2013. http://www.medscape.com/viewarticle/808930.

Mulcahy, Nick. "Online Nutritional Advice for Cancer Patients Is Scattershot."
Medscape.com, March 29, 2013. http://www.medscape.com/viewarticle/781706.

Nazaryan, Alexander. "World War Cancer." *The New Yorker,* June 2013.

Neergaard, Lauran. "Report Finds Aging U.S. Faces Crisis in Cancer Care." *The
Huffington Post*, September 10, 2013.
http://www.huffingtonpost.com/2013/09/10/cancer-care_n_3902356.html.

O: The Oprah Magazine. "The Best Way to Prevent Cancer: A Good Diet." *O: The
Oprah Magazine*, May 2010. http://www.oprah.com/health/Prevent-Cancer-with-
the-Right-Diet-of-Antiangiogenic-Foods/print/1.

Parker-Pope, Tara. "Medical Bills Cause Most Bankruptcies." *New York Times*, June 2009.
http://well.blogs.nytimes.com/2009/06/04/medical-bills-cause-most-bankruptcies/
comment-page-8/?_r=0.

Pecorino, Lauren. *Molecular Biology of Cancer: Mechanisms, Targets, and Therapeutics.*
Oxford, UK: Oxford University Press, 2012.

Prendergast, George C., Richard Metz, and Alexander J. Muller. "Towards a Genetic
Definition of Cancer-Associated Inflammation: Role of the IDO Pathway."
American Journal of Pathology, May 2010.

Ruiz, Don Miguel, MD. *The Four Agreements: A Practical Guide to Personal Freedom
(A Toltec Wisdom Book).* San Rafael, CA: Amber-Allen Publishing, 1997.

Sabin, Glenn. "Hospital Systems Ignore Integrative Medicine at Their Peril."
http://fonconsulting.com/uncategorized/hospital-systems-ignore-integrative-
medicine-at-their-peril/.

Servan-Schreiber, David, MD, PhD. *Anticancer: A New Way of Life.* New York: Viking, 2008.

Siegel, Bernie. *Love, Medicine and Miracles: Lessons Learned about Self-Healing from a Surgeon's Experience with Exceptional Patients.* New York: Harper & Row, 1986.

Society of Gynecologic Oncology. "More Than 60 Percent of Ovarian Cancer Patients Do Not Receive Recommended Treatment, Study Shows." *Society of Gynecologic Oncology*, March 2013. http://www.sgo.org/newsroom/news-releases/more-than-60-percent-of-ovarian-cancer-patients-do-not-receive-recommended-treatment/.

Tamkins, Theresa. "Medical Bills Prompt More Than 60 Percent of U.S. Bankruptcies." CNN.com, June 2009. http://www.cnn.com/2009/HEALTH/06/05/bankruptcy.medical.bills/index.html?_s=PM.

Thetford, William T. and Helen Schucman, eds. *A Course in Miracles.* Mill Valley, CA: The Foundation for Inner Peace, 1976.

Trent, Laura. "The State of Cancer Care in America, 2014: A Report by The American Society of Clinical Oncology." *Journal of Oncology Practice.* http://jop.ascopubs.org/content/10/2/119.full.

Turner, Kelly, PhD. *Radical Remission: Surviving Cancer Against All Odds.* New York: HarperCollins, 2014. http://www.drkellyturner.com/.

University of California – San Francisco. "Men with Prostate Cancer Should Eat Healthy Vegetable Fats, Study Suggests." *Science Daily*, June 10, 2013. http://www.sciencedaily.com/releases/2013/06/130610192948.htm.

U.S. News & World Report Health with Duke Medicine. "Personalized Health." *U.S. News & World Report Health.* http://health.usnews.com/health-conditions/cancer/personalized-medicine/overview.

Varona, Verne. *Nature's Cancer-Fighting Foods.* New York: Perigee, 2014.

Acknowledgments

Writing this book was not my idea early on. Around two and a half years into my diagnosis, a number of friends and colleagues encouraged me to journal about the experiences I was going through so that others might learn from them. A couple years later, when I was in a clinical trial at Columbia Presbyterian Hospital, my partner Kathleen and a number of my friends strongly encouraged me to document my story. Much of the groundwork and strategies in the book came through during my writing sessions while I was sitting in Central Park, resting between scans and tests. The past few years following my transplant in 2009 were spent compiling and sorting through the data and research I had collected.

I would like to start by acknowledging and thanking my partner Kathleen for her continuous love, caring, and support since we met many years ago. I could never repay her for the weeks, months, and years that she sacrificed her time, energy, and emotions to help save my life. She is the most wonderful, beautiful woman I have ever met. I am eternally grateful for her.

My mother has also been a critical lifeline in my survival. I cannot count the number of ways she has been a blessing to me. Her unconditional love, prayers, and support have lifted me up during my darkest hours. I want the world to know how much she has meant to me.

Next, I would like to give many thanks to the founder of Attitudinal Healing, Dr. Jerry Jampolsky, and his wife Dr. Diane Cirincione for their endless love and support during my fight for survival. I am very grateful to Jerry for his Attitudinal Healing Principles, which helped keep me alive. *Jerry and Diane, I will always be indebted to both of you for going above and beyond with your love and prayers. They have meant so much.* I also want to thank my Metro Detroit Center for Attitudinal Healing family for never leaving me in my time of need. Extra thanks go to cofounder Dr. Laurie Pappas, and her husband Ed for the myriad of ways in which they showed their love. I am deeply indebted to both of them. *Laurie, I will never forget the group healing sessions in your basement that helped keep me alive early on. Ed, I am very grateful for your time and expertise surrounding the business aspects of the book. I don't know how I can repay you and your partner.*

In 2007 I met Bob Clemente, the CEO of Behavioral Care Solutions, and I started to work for him as a clinician. During that time, I was undergoing chemo and only able to work part time. Whenever I became seriously ill, he always seemed to be there, bringing me food and visiting me in the hospital, while always encouraging me. Furthermore, he would often reassure me that I would have a job, no matter how much sick time I took off. This has been an enormous weight off my shoulders and has enabled me to always move forward. I'd like to thank author Dr. Spencer Johnson for his insight into the world of book publishing. *Your wonderful support and guidance were greatly appreciated. The time that you spent with me and Jerry meant so much to me.*

I'd like to thank writer, author, and screenwriter Mark Stein (via Terry Daru) for his wisdom and guidance during the last 18 months of this project. *I really appreciate the time that you've given me, you've helped the book immensely.*

I am very grateful for the help from my friend, Dr. Augustine Perrotta, an oncologist in Oakland County, Michigan, for reviewing my manuscript and his overall guidance. He is also a clinical professor of medicine emeritus at Michigan State University College of Medicine and author of the new book *A View from the Inside.*

Furthermore, I would like to thank Susan Thiem, the current executive director of the Metro Detroit Center for Attitudinal Healing, and her partner Gordon for their fundraising efforts and emotional support. *I am deeply grateful for your friendship over the decades. You have always given me love, emotional support, and wise counsel. Gordon, thank you for going above and beyond, driving me to and from Cleveland.* I also don't want to forget Ron and Linda Cohen for going above and beyond anything I could imagine. Their love and generosity know no bounds. *You've treated me like family, done so many favors, and put your lives on hold while you've accompanied me to Cleveland Clinic and other hospitals. Both of you have taken enormous stress off Kathleen and me countless times over the past decade.* Extra kudos to all the individuals acquainted with Attitudinal Healing who helped me with fundraising and other gifts.

Additionally, my deep gratitude goes to Rick Jones, JD, who is on the staff of the Dickinson Wright law firm. *Your wisdom and guidance has helped me enormously.*

I am very grateful to have Ilene Stankiewicz as my content and copy editor for this project. I don't know what I would have done without her. She went above and beyond anything I would have imagined to make this book an excellent read. I would highly recommend her to any author.

Kudos to Michelle Wallace from Cleveland, Ohio. She is a gifted writer and editor for whom I am deeply grateful. Her expertise in medical editing was very apparent to me. I appreciate her research efforts and summaries for the more difficult chapters.

I would like to thank Deborah Perdue, my graphic artist and book designer, for the wonderful work she did on this project. Kathleen and I are very appreciative of her time and her gifts that she gave. She is a wonderful guide and mentor.

I want to express my appreciation and gratitude to Cleveland Clinic in Cleveland, Ohio and their world-renowned liver transplant team. Dr. John Fung, Dr. Charles Miller, and Dr. Bijan Eghtesad played a crucial part in saving my life after so many had given up on me.

Dr. John Fung (liver transplant surgeon, Chairman of the Digestive Disease Institute)—*You were the original conduit and gatekeeper early on in allowing me to receive a liver transplant. Your worldwide reputation as a leader in transplant surgery speaks for itself. I am so fortunate to have had you by my side from the beginning.*

Dr. Bijan Eghtesad (my primary liver transplant surgeon)—*I am so grateful for the 13-hour transplant that you and your team performed. Not only are you a world-class transplant surgeon, you are a humble, kind, human being who continues to reassure me during my follow-up visits.*

Dr. Charles Miller (transplant surgeon, Director of Liver Transplantation in the Transplantation Center)—*I am very grateful that you vetted and approved me to receive a new liver. In addition, I want to thank you for your excellent care in the hospital.*

Dr. Cristiano Quintini (transplant surgeon)—*Thank you so much for using your excellent surgical skills during my transplant. Your expertise has allowed me to stay alive.*

Dr. Brian Rubin (sarcoma pathologist)—*Thank you for examining my slides. I am deeply grateful for your research towards the therapy for EHE.*

Jim Filisky and Rich Adams, Registered Nurses (liver transplant coordinators)—*I am deeply grateful for you helping me stay afloat after my transplant. I am so thankful for both of you going above and beyond when I had a health crisis. The care you give your patients is excellent.*

Cassie Gritzman, MSW—*Thank you for making my life less stressful each time I come to Cleveland Clinic. You seem to understand Kathleen's and my needs and what we have gone through. Thank you for your generosity.*

This acknowledgment could never express the deep sense of gratitude and appreciation that I have for the following clinicians and medical centers that saved my life:

Dr. Riad Salem, MD, MBA (Northwestern Memorial Hospital, Chicago, Illinois)—*I am so grateful for you keeping me alive while my vena cava was shutting down in my liver. The two procedures you performed on me went flawlessly and bought me time until my liver transplant. I will never forget what you did for me.*

Dr. Robert Taub, MD, PhD, and his sarcoma team (Columbia Presbyterian Medical Center, New York, New York)—*I am so grateful for your exceptional care and willingness to accept me into your Sutent® Trial, which kept me alive from 2006-2009, until my transplant. You did this and so much more for me. The "fatherly" concern and guidance meant as much to me as the treatment.*

Dr. Scott Schwartz (Henry Ford Medical Center, Detroit, Michigan)—*Dr. Scott, you literally saved my life. I highly recommend you to anyone needing interventional radiology. Your expertise in the field of hepatic oncology is outstanding.*

Dr. Sheela Tejwani (Henry Ford Medical Center, Detroit, Michigan)—*Thank you for your care and surveillance since my transplant. I really appreciate the thoroughness of your approach. Furthermore, I am thankful that you are an open-minded, eclectic clinician who can think outside the box. I am grateful to be in your hands.*

Dr. Thomas Doyle (Henry Ford Medical Center, Detroit, Michigan)—
Thank you so much for your excellent care before my transplant.

Jeff McMahon, PA-C (physician assistant, Henry Ford Medical Center,
Detroit, Michigan)—*Thank you for your skilled expertise at performing
numerous procedures while I was in liver failure. I appreciated your calm, soothing
manner during desperate times.*

Dr. Helen Lee, MD, integrative clinician, and staff (Farmington
Medical Center, Farmington Hills, Michigan)—When most of my
other doctors had given up on or had left me, she was there.
*You always had time for me, were constantly researching my case, trou-
bleshooting my problems, and filling in the gaps to assure my survival.
I am deeply grateful.*

Beaumont Hospital Emergency Medicine (Royal Oak, Michigan)—*I'd
like to thank the physicians, mid-level clinicians, and staff for your excellent care
during the many times I have come there for help. Your expertise and attention to
detail helped minimize my side effects and complications.*

Dr. Scott Silver (William Beaumont Hospital, Royal Oak, Michigan)—
*Thank you so much for your excellent care during and after my blood clot
experience. The time you spend with me, showing me the nuances of my DVT,
has been invaluable.*

Dr. Russell Steinman (William Beaumont Hospital, Royal Oak,
Michigan)—*Thank you for taking care of my heart with all its post chemo issues and complications. The ablation that you performed relieved a lot of my
stress. I am very grateful.*

Dr. Joel Kahn (clinical professor of medicine, Wayne State University School of Medicine and Director of Cardiac Wellness, Michigan Healthcare Professionals, PC)—*Thank you for your wonderful care and teaching me about integrative cardiology. Your guidance has helped abate my cardiac complications from the chemo.*

Dr. Myron Schwartz (liver transplant surgeon, Mount Sinai Medical Center, New York, New York)—*I want to thank you for the many times over the years that you gave me your expertise and advice during critical periods of my survival.*

Vascular Anomalies Center, Boston Children's Hospital, founded by the late Dr. Judah Folkman (Boston, Massachusetts)—*I am deeply grateful for your research and assistance regarding my tumor. The information you gave me was valuable and your guidance was superb.*

Dr. Michael Harbut (Detroit Medical Center)—*I am extremely grateful for the many times that you guided me through very difficult medical decisions. It's comforting to know that your wise counsel is always at hand.*

Dr. Ferre Akbarpour (Chief Medical Officer, Orange County Immune Institute, Huntington Beach, California)—*Thank you so much for being one of the first medical professionals to give me hope during the early spring of 2004. Your integrative treatments were immensely helpful.*

Dr. Robert LaCoste (Crittendon Hospital and Behavioral Care Solutions, Rochester, Michigan)—*Thank you for your tutoring, guidance, and friendship. I also want to give thanks for your fundraising efforts that helped pay my medical expenses.*

Dr. Marc Liebeskind (radiologist, New York, New York)—*I want to tell you how much I appreciated your skills and expertise during my illness. I also give thanks for your willingness to always be accessible to me.*

Dr. Robert Schwert (oncologist, Traverse City, Michigan)—*Thank you for helping to keep me alive early on.*

The following people supported me in researching and/or compiling my book manuscript. Early on, I was lucky enough to have met writing coach Jeannie Ballew, owner of Edit Prose (Ann Arbor, Michigan), who is a very gifted writer. Her skill set and talent have improved my original manuscript tremendously. I could not have completed it without her. Kathryn Curtis (Kat) also supplied excellent research to flesh out my chapters. Cancer survivor Elyn Jacobs helped enormously with her expertise and research concerning the anticancer nutrition chapter, and she interviewed me on her radio show *Survive and Live Well.*

My close friend, Bronni Fogg (an IT specialist), and her husband Richard were invaluable in guiding me as I sifted through data and revised the chapters. They both spent many weeks and months helping to put this book together. I am deeply indebted to them both.

Kudos to our friend, Debra Henning, who is a gifted teacher and possible beginning editor. *The time you spent editing and reviewing the manuscript has been invaluable. Furthermore, your gourmet, homemade meals certainly helped me to heal.*

My deepest gratitude also goes out to my church family (Church of the Holy City), especially to my minister Renee, and Joe Michiniak. *Renee, the healing you both did for me and continue to do has meant so much. I will never forget when you came to visit me in Cleveland after my transplant. It was a rough time, but having you there made all the difference. Kathleen and I have been so grateful for your ongoing support and friendship.* Special thanks goes to Theron Cromwell, retired minister at my church, who drove me in the middle of the night to Cleveland for my transplant. Moreover, he kept me company for weeks and played chess with me to help relieve some of the stress of the ordeal. Peg Lindsey also helped Kathleen and me in many ways, including with meals and extra nurturing. Lastly, I want to thank Nancy and Charlie Gehringer for their outpouring of kindness and support. *When we were too tired and stressed to cook for ourselves, your dinner invitations meant so much. Kathleen and I are so very grateful.*

I would like to thank two wonderfully gifted spiritual directors at the Manresa Jesuit Retreat Center in Bloomfield Hills, Michigan, Mary McKeon and Paula Dow, who lifted me from the depths of despair while I was fighting for my life. Furthermore, they have given generously of their time and have prayed with me repeatedly over the past six years. They gave me hope where there was none.

My gratitude also goes out to Theresa Turnbull, RN, and her fiancé Allen Shaw, a couple who have stood by me and given me unconditional love and acceptance since the beginning of this journey. I will never forget all the little (and *big*) things that they have both done over the past decade. *You both have been a continuing lifeline to me in so many ways. Allen, your savvy listening skills and advice have been invaluable. Your visit to me in the days following my transplant meant so much.*

My thanks also go out to my buddies, including my college friend, Steve Kanuiga. Steve was there at my beside in the ICU after my transplant. I can never repay him for all he has done for me, both before and after the surgery. *Steve, I plan on using your excellent marketing and artistic skills following the launch of this book.* Kudos also go to Larry Vergeldt and Adam Beyer for standing by me and always giving me their best.

I also want to thank my dad Lynn; my sister, Anne, and her husband Ken; and my sister, Pam, and her husband Mike for their help, especially early on. My gratitude also goes out to my Uncle Johnny and Aunt Meg Wonser for their prayers and letters of support.

Michelle Phaump, founder of Lend a Helping Hand; Dr. Martin Brown; Mike Coraci, PA; Jim Tuman; Michael Wickett; and Howard Kaplan also have my undying gratitude for all of the fundraising they did, along with spiritual and emotional support. *Your help relieved my financial burdens enormously.*

I'd like to thank the Reverend Chuck Hancock and his wife Lois for organizing the prayer event for me at Unity Church in Royal Oak, Michigan. Additionally, I'd like to thank you for your support and fundraising efforts over the past 12 years. *Your love and concern have meant so much.*

Speaking of fundraisers, I'd like to acknowledge Chris and Kelly Burek, Susie and Dave Brice, Karen and Jacques Ledent, Dr. John Kamar, and Jerry and LaVonne Parsh for their love and support in attending the 2008-2009 fundraisers for my benefit.

I would also like to express my gratitude for the caring animals in my life, cats Zsa Zsa and Cubey. Both of them spent months, even years, sending me their positive energy by lying on and purring over my liver and relieving my pain and suffering.

My Internet support group Hemangioendothelioma (HE), Epithelioid Hemangioendothelioma (EHE), and Related Vascular Disorders (HEARD) were and have been critical in my survival. Members Avi and Lila Dogim have been my angels many times over, connecting me with Dr. Robert Taub at Columbia Presbyterian Hospital and letting me stay at their condo on the Hudson River in New Jersey while I was in clinical trials. I so appreciate their generosity. I'd also like to thank HEARD member Dr. Guy Weinberg, professor of anesthesiology at Chicago Medical Center, for his wonderful guidance and expertise throughout my illness. It has meant so much to me.

Additionally, I want to thank Jane Gutkovich, the mother of a fellow EHE survivor. *Your tireless research and advocacy has meant so much to me and other EHE survivors. I hope to work with you more closely in the future.*